MEDICAL TERMINOLOGY:

An Innovative and Successful Approach

Charles A. Henderson, MD
Lauren F. Liddell

MedTutor.com

MedTutor.com

1501 S. 40th Avenue
Hattiesburg, MS 39402

Cover: Bice Advertising, Inc.

Typesetting and Page Layout: Jan D. Lacy, Copy Cats Printing, Inc.

Medical Terminology: An Innovative and Successful Approach

ISBN# 978-0-9827485-2-7

Printed in the United States of America.

To God and the
beauty of His creation.

Contents

CONTENTS

Introduction

"Whatever you can do, or dream you can do, begin it.
Boldness has genius, power, and magic in it."

– Johann Wolfgang von Goethe

INTRO

Much of the challenge associated with pursuing a medical-related education and subsequent career can be linked to a lack of familiarity with medical language. There is a seemingly inexhaustible number of terms not known by the lay public that routinely appear in the performance of a medical job. The sooner an individual becomes familiar with this terminology, the sooner he or she can excel in the classroom or workplace.

Language is not only a mechanism for communication. It is also an important tool for thought. Someone with a superior vocabulary is not only able to describe situations more concisely, he or she can also think in a more precise and efficient manner.

Thousands pursue medical careers each year, yet few are familiar with medical terminology at the start of their new job or school. Relying on the random exposure to individual terms during daily activities is a very inefficient way to improve one's knowledge of medical terminology. Yet with so many terminology books available, one has to wonder why more people are not better prepared.

There are several reasons for this deficiency. First and foremost, most people are intimidated and overwhelmed by the magnitude of information. It appears that there is simply too much information to learn by self-study. To actually learn medical terminology systematically is a daunting task. Additionally, attempting to master terminology by merely reading a regular medical vocabulary text is analogous to attempting to learn English by reading a dictionary. The material in these texts is often boring and difficult to study for any significant duration. Although the meanings of certain terms may indeed be interesting, the monotonous task of studying one word definition after another can quickly drive the mind to wander.

Instead of attempting to teach each individual word, this text concentrates on explaining Greek and Latin word combining forms. This approach is taken because many of the English medical terms are derived from Greek and Latin prefixes, word roots, and suffixes. Medical terms are "built" by combining these Greek and Latin word forms.

A prefix is one or more syllables placed in front of a word to modify its meaning. Even the word "prefix" demonstrates this since "pre" is Latin for "before." Some other common examples of prefixes include *an-, bi-, di-, para-,* and *sub-*. A word root is the base component of a word; it denotes the subject of the word. In the word "prefix," "fix" is the word root. It is Latin for "to fasten." Thus "prefix" as a whole means "to fasten before." Some examples of medical word roots are the root for the liver, *hepat-*, and the root for the nose, *rhino-*. Finally, a suffix is one or more syllables placed at the back of a word to modify its meaning. A few examples of common suffixes found in medical terminology are -cele, -ducent, -gram, -mittent, and -oid.

If the meanings of the various components contained in an unknown medical term are known, the meaning of the whole term becomes apparent. The value of this cannot be stressed enough. Once the reader learns the combining forms, he or she will be able to deduce the meaning of many unfamiliar medical words that have never been seen before. A whole new language will be unlocked. Additionally, because the name of a medical term becomes logically evident in this process, the word itself is much easier to remember.

Consider the example of paranephritis. A person with knowledge of medical combining forms could make an educated guess at the meaning, even if the word had never been seen or heard before. The prefix, *para-*, means *beside*. For example, a *para*site lives on or within (*beside*) another living organism and the *para*sympathetic nervous system is *beside* the sympathetic nervous system. *Nephr-* is a word root for *kidney*. Thus a *nephr*ologist is a physician who specializes in the treatment of *kidney* disorders and a *nephr*on is the basic structural unit of the *kidney*. Finally, *-itis* is a suffix that denotes *inflammation*. Appendic*itis* is *inflammation* of the appendix. Pharyng*itis* is *inflammation* of structures of the pharynx. Thus, place the meanings of the prefix (*para-*), word root (*nephr-*), and suffix (*-itis*) together and one can assume that "paranephritis" is an inflammation of tissues near the kidney.

The key to unlocking medical language is found in the two-tiered system that is encompassed by this book and the two interactive *courses* found on its associated website, **Medtutor.com**. Attention in the first course is directed at learning medical combining forms. This is accomplished by studying the book first and then accessing the website to participate in the web-based learning applications of the *medical combining forms course*. These interactive applications provide a fun method of exposure to combining forms and include randomized exams, flashcards, and medical crossword puzzles. When the student feels confident in his or her knowledge, a final exam on combining forms can be taken on the website.

At this point, the student should be well-acquainted with many combining forms and can then participate in the second tier of the system, the *medical terminology course*. This course contains the same three interactive applications as the combining form course and introduces the student to thousands of new medical terms.

Medical terms identified in the online applications are categorically linked to particular medical specialties such as pediatrics, cardiology, or dentistry. Exam questions and flashcards may be selected and viewed based on a medical specialty or any combination of specialties. In each learning application, the student attempts to deduce the meaning of the term based on its components. The term is then defined and all combining form components that are contained in the word are reviewed. The student thus obtains the dual benefit of learning medical terminology while also becoming an expert in medical combining forms.

BOOK

The book is divided into six chapters, including this introductory chapter, four chapters that focus on medical combining forms, and a conclusion that contains information on the use and navigation of the website. There is one chapter for each of the three types of combining forms: prefixes, word roots, and suffixes. The combining forms are placed in alphabetical order in each of these three chapters. Chapter five is composed of a random assortment of all combining forms covered in the previous three.

The page layout is similar in the four chapters that contain combining forms. Each page is formed by three columns. The word combining forms create a column on the left side of the page. The definitions of the combining forms comprise a second column in the middle of the page. Finally, examples of the use of each combining form make up a third column on the right side of the page.

As an effective study mechanism, the reader can use a folded sheet of paper or card to cover the two columns on the right, leaving the word combining forms in the left-sided column as the only ones visible. After consideration, the paper can be slid to the right to reveal the meaning of a particular combining form.

Even if the correct definition was not initially known, the reader should attempt to think of examples of the use of the combining form in everyday language and then move on to study the examples in the third column. This process will highly facilitate learning and memorization.

Chapter Five provides a second, random exposure to each combining form. Here, prefixes, suffixes, and word roots are randomly listed without regard to alphabetical order. The reader should progress through the chapter in the same manner as described above. Upon completing these chapters, the student will be familiar enough with the combining forms to participate in the internet applications and training programs.

WEB-BASED INTERACTIVE LEARNING APPLICATIONS

The website contains an array of interactive applications for the various *Medtutor* books that exist. The customizable applications allow the student to direct the system as to which books (courses) or book chapters to pull information from. The applications are designed to provide a unique, efficient, and effective mechanism for enhancing learning. The website also tracks the individual student's progress, allowing him or her to tailor the exercises to focus on particular problem areas. Available applications include randomized examinations, flashcards, medical crossword puzzles, interactive posters, and final examinations. In addition to being viewable on conventional computers, *Medtutor* applications are also designed to be compatible for use with mobile devices.

RANDOMIZED EXAM APPLICATION

The randomized exam system includes a database of thousands of questions related to combining forms and medical terminology. This system is incredibly dynamic, flexible and customizable. At any time, the student can prompt the system to assimilate a test composed of a certain number of randomized questions. This exam may contain questions specific to a particular combining form chapter, to a group of chapters, or to the entire book. The questions may be limited to a certain medical specialty or any combination of specialties. The exams may also be tailored to contain questions from both terminology courses (medical combining forms and medical terminology) or can even be designed to comprise a mixture from other *Medtutor* books and their chapters. Furthermore, the student can also direct the system to assemble exams solely from questions the student has never seen before, questions previously passed, those previously failed, or a combination of all question subgroups.

Every exam is timed and automatically graded. Answers and detailed explanations are provided upon completion. Each question is categorized to the specific combining form category or to the area of medicine it applies. The system displays the number of questions and percentage correct for each of the various subdivisions. Problem areas can be identified and future exams can be created to target those areas.

To facilitate tracking, a progress bar and a score bar are provided for each group of questions that are associated with each chapter or category. This allows the student to instantaneously know where he or she currently stands in each category of information at any given time. Out of the total number of questions that are available for a particular chapter or category, the system displays the percentage of questions that have previously been seen by the student. This percentage is displayed as a *progress* bar. Out of the questions that have previously been seen by the student, the system also displays the percentage that were answered correctly. This is displayed as a *score* bar. The student may then tailor future exercises to focus on particular problem areas.

FLASHCARDS

The flashcard application also possesses dynamic and customizable properties. The database associated with the medical combining form course contains one card for every combining form in this book. On the front side of the card is the name of the word combining form. The back contains its meaning and examples of its use. The user directs the system as to the number and type of flashcards to display during a particular sitting. Like the questions that appear in a randomized exam, flashcards may be studied based on a specific combining form chapter, group of chapters, or the entire book.

The front of each card in the second course, the medical terminology course, contains a medical term. If prompted, an audio application will provide the correct pronunciation of the term. The back of the card displays the definition of the word and reviews the meanings of each of the combining form components that are contained in the term. Medical terminology flashcards may be studied based on medical specialty and can be combined with cards from the medical combining form course or other *Medtutor* books and their chapters.

Upon completion of a particular set of cards, the

student may prompt the system to display the same set of cards backwards in order to show the back of each card first. Alternatively, the user may direct the system to initially present the back of each card from the onset. The student has the ability to pass or fail him/herself on each flashcard. Failed flashcards are placed in a personalized databank that can be accessed and reviewed at any time. Cards that are subsequently marked as "passed" are removed from the databank; "failed" cards remain. The personalized format of the randomized exam and flashcard applications allows the student to efficiently navigate an immense amount of information.

CROSSWORD PUZZLES

The medical crossword puzzles are an informal way to continually review and learn new material. The system can be directed to create a puzzle specific to information contained in either of the two courses associated with this book or some combination of other *Medtutor* books. If a crossword question is not known, the application provides a short explanation when requested. All crossword puzzles can be worked online or printed and worked while away from the computer. The student can return to the internet site at any time to check answers and obtain explanations.

As with the other applications, the crossword puzzle application can be integrated to include information across multiple courses. Since there is a significant amount of fundamental medical information presented in the *Medtutor* series, even working just one puzzle a day would greatly benefit any practitioner in a health-related profession.

WEB-BASED FINAL EXAMS

After sufficient preparation, the student can go to the website and take the final exam for each of the two terminology courses (medical combining forms and medical terminology). Each examination mimics a board-type exam and contains 180 questions divided into two 90 question segments. The student has three hours to take each exam and a break is provided between the two segments. The final exams may seem long, but each is designed to mimic a board-type exam, in which mental fatigue plays a role. The test is immediately graded and answers and explanations are provided. Each question is categorized so the student knows how well he or she did in a given category. Students who answer more than 70% of questions correctly are considered to have passed. As designated by the student, the website can then e-mail a letter of score verification to relatives, teachers, organizations, or the admissions offices of schools or course programs. This can be done for either or both exams, and it serves as a testimony of your motivation and hard work.

The path to success is in front of you. Perseverance is the key. The process is simple, but it is not easy. The book is not merely meant to be read, but to actively be *engaged.* Short-term and long-term goals should be employed to ensure that a meaningful amount is learned by a particular date. The type of studying may be quite different than that which you have previously performed. Go slow and be certain that the material is learned before moving on. Avoid trying to accomplish too much in one sitting to help you retain what you learn. Whenever a study session is completed, set a date for when your next session will occur and adhere to it. There are over 900 combining forms in this book. If the student learns ten a day, it will take ninety days to learn them all. If a student learns twenty a day, the material can be learned in half that time. Find the pace that is most effective for you and stick to it.

The book serves as a convenient and portable mechanism to study. The web-based applications provide a unique and fun way to accelerate and reinforce the learning process. Much will be gained by completing the course and continuing to participate in the web-based applications on a regular basis. Again, a competency in medical language will equip you with significant advantages over others who have not made an effort to become medically fluent. *Good luck.*

– Charles A. Henderson, MD

Medical Prefixes

"Always bear in mind that your own resolution to succeed is more important than any other."

– Abraham Lincoln

PREFIXES

MEDICAL PREFIX	MEANING	EXAMPLES
a(n)-	not; without	**a**febrile – Without fever.
		analgesia – Without pain.
ab-	away from	**ab**duct – A motion in which a structure is moved away from the midline of the body.
		abrasion – Tissue is scraped away from the skin or mucous membrane.
ac-	to; add	**ac**cumulation – To add onto or build up.
		accustom – To become familiar with.
ad-	to, when not preceding the consonants *c,f,g,p,s,* or *t*	**ad**duct – Movement toward the midline of a structure. To adduct the arm is to bring it down the side of the body. To adduct the fingers is to bring them together so they are closer to the midline of the upper extremity.
		adneural – Toward a nerve (as electric current passes from muscle to nerve).
allo-	other; different	**allo**rhythmia – Having an irregular heartbeat.
		allosome – A foreign part of the cytoplasm in a cell that entered from the outside.
ambi-	both; around	**ambi**dextrous – Can use either hand well.
		ambient temperature – The surrounding temperature.
ambo-	both	**ambo**n – The cartilaginous ring around a bone socket containing the head of a long bone.
		amboceptor – The double receptor of hemolysin.
amphi-	both; both sides	**amphi**arthrosis – A joint attached on both sides by fibrocartilage, allowing little motion and providing strength.
		amphibians – Vertebrates that can live both in water and on land.
an-	without; not	**an**oxia – Without oxygen.
		anesthesia – The loss of sensation.

MEDICAL PREFIX	MEANING	EXAMPLES
ana-	upward; backward, again, excessive	**ana**bolism – A building process where simple substances are converted to more complex compounds.
		anaplasia – Cells begin to grow in a more primitive pattern.
ante-	forward	**ante**rior – A direction or location toward the front (opposite of posterior).
		antenna – One of the two forward appendages on the head of arthropods.
antero-	in front of	**antero**grade – Moving or extending forward.
		anterolateral – A direction toward or location in the front and to one side.
anti-	counteractive; against	**anti**dote – An agent or mechanism that counteracts a poison.
		antiemetic – An agent or mechanism that relieves or prevents nausea.
apo-	separation; derived from	**apo**protein – The protein portion of a molecule.
		apophysis – An outgrowth. Often used to describe bony outgrowths that do not separate from the bone (e.g. tubercle process).
as-	to, when preceding the consonant *s*	**as**similate – take in and understand; absorb and digest.
atre-	closed	biliary **atre**sia – Lack or obliteration of the bile duct.
auto-	self	**auto**immunity – An immune response against tissues of the patient's own body.
		autotransfusion – Transfusion of the patient's own blood.
bacill-	rod-like	**bacill**us – A genus of rod-shaped bacteria.
		bacilliform – Having a rod-shaped form.
bas-	base	**bas**ophil – Readily stained with basic dyes.
		basilad – Toward the base.
bathy-	deep	**bathy**pnea – To breathe deeply.

MEDICAL PREFIXES

MEDICAL PREFIX	MEANING	EXAMPLES
bi-	two	**bi**lateral – Both sides.
		bicep – A muscle with two points of origin.
bili-	bile	**bili**rubin – A bile pigment.
		biliary atresia – Lack or obliteration of the bile duct.
bis-	twice	**bis**albuminemia – A condition in which two types of albumin are present in an individual.
		bisiliac – Associated with the two iliac bones.
blenn-	mucus	**blenn**orrhea – The discharge or mucus.
brady-	slow	**brady**cardia – Slowing of the heart rate.
		bradypnea – Abnormal slowness of breath.
brevi-	short	**brevi**collis – Shortness of the neck.
		brevirostrate – A short beak.
cac-	abnormal	**cac**hexia – State of ill health and malnutrition.
		cacogeusia – A bad taste not associated with something ingested.
cata-	negative; against; down	**cata**bolism – The breaking down of complex substances into more simple substances.
		catagen – A portion of the hair cycle in which growth stops.
cav-	hollow	**cav**ernous – Pertaining to or associated with a hollow space.
		cavity – A hollow place inside the body.
cen-	common	**cen**esthesia – The general feeling of the presence of one's own body.
centr-	center	**centr**iciput – The center portion of the upper surface of the head.
		centripetal – Toward a center.
cheil-	lip	**cheil**oschisis – A split lip; harelip.
		cheilitis – Inflammation of the lips.

MEDICAL PREFIX	MEANING	EXAMPLES
chir-	hand; also spelled cheir-	**chir**oplasty – Plastic surgery on the hand.
		chiromegaly – Enlargement of the hands.
chlor-	green	**chlor**ophyll – A green pigment found in plants.
		chloroma – A malignant tumor that is green in color.
choan-	funnel	**choan**oid – Funnel-shaped.
		choana – An opening into the nasopharynx of the nasal cavity.
cili-	eyelids	**cili**ary – Associated with or pertaining to the eye and its surrounding structures.
		ciliectomy – Surgical excision of part of the eyelid.
circu-	around	**circu**mcision – Removal of the skin that wraps around the tip of the penis.
		circulation – Movement of blood throughout the body.
cis-	same side	**cis**platin – A platinum complex used to create interstrand DNA crosslinks.
clus-	shut	in**clus**ion – The act of closing; being closed.
		oc**clus**ion – Obstruction; trapped liquids or gases; relation of teeth on each jaw when in contact; closure of some area of the vocal tract.
co-	with; together	**co**hesion – The intermolecular force which causes particles of a material to unite.
		cohort – A group of individuals sharing a common characteristic.
coel-	hollow	**coel**om – Body cavity.
		coelozoic – Living in the intestinal canal of the body.
coll-	glue	**coll**ide – To crash into one another.
		collagen – The major protein component of connective tissue.

MEDICAL PREFIX	MEANING	EXAMPLES
com-	with; together	**com**mensalism – A relationship between two organisms in which one benefits while the other is unaffected.
		compound – Made up of two or more parts.
con-	with; together	**con**nect – To put together.
		contagious – The ability of a disease to be transferred to another.
contra-	opposite; against	**contra**rian – An individual who opposes the position taken by the majority.
		contralateral – Affecting the opposite side.
corpor-	body	**corpor**ation – A group of people that act as one body.
cox-	hip	**cox**algia – Pain in the hip.
		coxa – The hip.
cune-	wedge	**cune**iform – Wedge-shaped.
		cuneus – Wedge-shaped segment on the medial aspect of the occipital lobe of the cerebrum.
de-	down; lack of	**de**compression – To remove pressure.
		degeneration – Going to higher to lower; declining.
deuter-	second	**deuter**anomaly – Most common color vision deficiency in which the second green-sensitive cones have decreased sensitivity.
		deuteropathy – Disease that is secondary to another disease.
di-	two; double	**di**ataxia – Loss of coordination of muscles on both sides of the body.
		diarthric – Pertaining to or affecting two different joints.
dia-	apart; through; between; complete	**dia**meter – The distance through the center of a circle.
		diarrhea – The flowing through of watery feces.

MEDICAL PREFIX	MEANING	EXAMPLES
dif-	apart; not	**dif**ficult – Not easy.
		diffraction – The spreading apart of light.
digit-	finger; toe	**digit**al – Performed with the fingers.
		inter**digit**ate – To weave or interlock like fingers do when holding hands.
dis-	apart; not	**dis**locate – To take apart or put out of place.
		disability – Not able to function normally.
dolich-	long	**dolich**ocephalic – Long headed.
dys-	bad; improper; difficult	**dys**function – Not working correctly.
		dyslexia – The inability to read, spell, and write words correctly.
e-	out from	**e**motion – A strong feeling state directed toward a specific object.
		emission – Discharge.
ec-	out of; outside	**ec**centric – Outside of the norm; a person who acts outside of normal character.
		ectopic – Not in the normal position.
ecto-	outside	**ecto**derm – In a developing embryo, the outermost germ layer.
		ectopia – Displacement of an organ or body part from its normal position.
ede-	swelling	**ede**ma – Swelling due to build up of fluid.
		edemagen – Something that causes edema.
ef-	out of; from	**ef**ferent – Going away from an organ or part.
		effusion – The escape of fluid; pouring out of.
electro-	amber; electrical	**electro**encephalography – Recording of changes in electric potential in various parts of the brain.
		electrolysis – Destruction by electromagnetic current.

MEDICAL PREFIXES

MEDICAL PREFIX	MEANING	EXAMPLES
em-	in; on	**em**bedding – To fix into something.
		emphysema – A condition caused by build up of air in tissues or organs.
en-	in; on	**en**clave – An area or group that is isolated within a larger one.
		endaural – Within the ear.
endo-	inside	**endo**derm – The innermost germ layer of the embryo.
		endometrium – The lining within the uterus.
ent-	inside	**ent**oblast – Endoderm.
		entoptic – Originating from within the eye.
epi-	after; upon; in addition to	**epi**dural – Located on the dura mater.
		epidermis – The outer layer of skin.
eryth-	red	**eryth**ematous – Redness of the skin, inflammation.
eso-	inside; within	**eso**tropia – Cross-eyed; when one eye turns inward towards the other eye.
eu-	good; normal; easy	**eu**pepsia – Good or normal digestion.
		euthanasia – A painless or easy death.
eury-	wide	**eury**cephalic – Having a wide head.
		euryon – A point on the parietal bone of the skull marking the greatest transverse diameter of the skull.
ex-	out of; away	**ex**cavation – To hollow out.
		excise – To take out by cutting.
exo-	outside	**exo**skeleton – An outer covering.
		exocrine – Secretion of hormones outside via a duct.

MEDICAL PREFIX	MEANING	EXAMPLES
extra-	outside of; beyond	**extra**terrestrial – Located outside of the earth.
		extrarenal – Located outside of the kidney.
fil-	thread-like	**fil**ament – A fiber or thread.
		filaria – A nematode worm.
fiss-	split	**fiss**ure – Any cleft or groove.
		fissula – Small cleft.
flav-	yellow	**flav**in – Water soluble yellow pigments that are diverse in animals and plants.
		***Flav**obacterium* – Genus of gram-negative, aerobic or facultatively anaerobic, soil and water bacteria which are characterized by the yellow pigment they produce.
gemin-	twin	**gemin**ate – Paired.
		geminal – Substituent atoms or groups attached to the same atom in a molecule.
geo-	Pertaining to earth or the Earth	**geo**medicine – Study of environmental and climatic effects on health.
		geophagia – Habitual eating of earth or clay.
hapl-	single	**hapl**oid – Having a single set of chromosomes.
hemi-	half	**hemi**sphere – Half of a globe or sphere. Also, half of the cerebrum or cerebellum.
		hemiplegia – Paralysis of one half of the body.
holo-	entire	**holo**enzyme – The entire enzyme composed of the coenzyme and apoenzyme.
homo-	like; same	**homo**type – One part having reversed symmetry with its pair (e.g. hands).
		homogenous – Made up of the same substances or parts.
hyper-	beyond; above	**hyper**emesis – Excessive vomiting.
		hyperglycemia – Elevated blood sugar level.

MEDICAL PREFIX	MEANING	EXAMPLES
hygr-	wet	**hygr**oma – Fluid-filled sac,cyst, or bursa.
		hygrometry – Measurement of moisture in the atmosphere.
hyp-	beneath; below; under	**hypo**dermic – Below the skin.
		hypoglycemia – An abnormally low blood glucose level.
		hypaxial – Ventral to the long axis of the body.
il-	not; within	**il**legible – Not clear enough to be read.
		illusion – Mental impression of reality which deviates from the actual event.
im-	not; within	**im**mature – Not fully developed.
		immersion – To dip something into a liquid.
in-	not; within	**in**adequate – Not adequate.
		incision – To cut into.
infra-	below; beneath; under	**infra**structure – The basic framework; foundation.
		infrasonic – Frequency that is below the range of hearing.
inter-	among; between	**inter**nal – Found on the inside.
		interaction – Action between individuals or substances.
intra-	inside; within	**intra**venous – Inside a vein.
		intracellular – Within a cell or cells.
intro-	within; into	**intro**spection – To look within.
		introvert – A person who keeps to themselves; to turn inward.
ipsi-	self; same	**ipsi**lateral – Associated with the same side of the body.
ir-	not; within	**ir**rational – Not rational.
		irradiation – To expose to radiation; to put rays into.

MEDICAL PREFIX	MEANING	EXAMPLES
iso-	equal	**iso**phoria – Equal tension of the vertical muscles in each eye.
		isochromatic – Equal or same color throughout.
juxta-	near; beside	**juxta**position – Side by side.
loc-	place	**loc**ator – Device used for determining the site of foreign objects in the body.
		trans**loc**ation – Movement of a substance from one site to another.
lyo-	loose; dissolve	**lyo**philic – Stable in solution.
		lyophobic – Unstable in solution.
macro-	large; long	**macro**melia – Having one or more limbs that are enlarged.
		macropsia – A visual disorder that causes objects to appear larger than they actually are.
mal-	bad	**mal**evolent – To wish evil on someone.
		malformation – A bad or faulty formation.
mani-	mental aberration	**mani**ac – Individual exhibiting characteristics of extreme or wild behavior.
medi-	middle	**medi**an – Situated in the midline of a body or structure.
mega-	large; great	**mega**logastria – An abnormally large stomach.
		megacystis – An enlarged bladder.
meta-	after; beyond; change	**meta**basis – The change in course of a disease.
		metapneumonic – To follow pneumonia.
mne-	pertaining to memory	a**mne**sia – Memory loss.
		mnemonic – Special technique used to improve memory.
mono-	only; single; solo	**mono**cular – Having only one eye.
		monochromatic – Having only one color.

MEDICAL PREFIXES

MEDICAL PREFIX	MEANING	EXAMPLES
multi-	many; much	**multi**para – A woman who has had two or more pregnancies.
		multinodular – Having many nodules.
nemat-	thread; thin	**nemat**ode – Roundworm.
neo-	new; young	**neo**natal – Pertaining to a newborn child.
		neoplasm – A new and abnormal growth.
non-	not	**non**disjunction – Failure of chromosomes to separate correctly.
		nonspecific – Not having a known cause.
noto-	pertaining to the back	**noto**chord – A rod-shaped system of cells on the dorsal aspect of an embryo serving, as the center for the development of the skeletal system.
nulli-	none	**nulli**para – A woman who has never given birth to a child.
		nullify – To make void.
ob-	against	**ob**tusion – Deadening of sensitiveness.
		obstruction – A blockage.
oc-	against	**oc**clusion – A blockage; trapping of liquid or gas within cavities; Relation of the teeth when in contact; momentary closure of the vocal tract.
		occult – Obscure; hidden.
omni-	every; all	**omni**potent – Having all power.
		omnivore – A person or animal that eats all kinds of foods.
omo-	shoulder	**omo**clavicular – Pertaining to the shoulder and the clavicle.
		omohyoid – Pertaining to the shoulder and the hyoid bone.
oscill-	back and forth	**oscill**ate – To move backward and forward like a spring or pendulum.
		oscillopsia – The visual illusion that objects are swaying back and forth.

MEDICAL PREFIX	MEANING	EXAMPLES
ossi-	bone	**ossi**ferous – Producing bone.
		ossicle – A small bone.
paleo-	old	**pale**ocortex – Portion of the cerebral cortex that develops with the olfactory system and is phylogenetically older than the neocortex.
		paleopathology – Study of diseases in bodies that have been preserved since ancient times.
palin-	recurring	**palin**dromia – Happening again.
		palinopsia – Preservation of a visual sensation after the stimulus is gone.
pan-	all	**pan**demic – Universal; a disease found throughout.
		pancytopenia – A lack of all blood cells.
para-	adjacent; beyond	**para**nasal – Adjacent to the nose.
		paranormal – Beyond scientific explanation.
pauci-	few	**pauci**synaptic – Involving only a few synapses in series.
pec-	fix; fasten	**pec**tin – Gelatinous polysaccharide that is present in fruits.
per-	through	**per**cutaneous – Given through or by way of the skin.
		peroral – Given through the mouth.
peri-	around	**peri**phery – The outward surface of a body.
		perimeter – The border or boundary of an area.
pero-	injured	**pero**melia – Severe anomaly of a limb or limbs resulting from embryonic development.
phall-	penis	**phall**oplasty – Plastic surgery of the penis.
		phallitis – Inflammation of the penis.
phleg-	burn	**phleg**masia – Inflammation.

MEDICAL PREFIXES

MEDICAL PREFIX	MEANING	EXAMPLES
phos-	light	**phos**e – Any visual stimulus such as light or color.
platy-	broad; flat	**platy**podia – Flat-footed.
		platyhelminthes – Flatworms.
pleo-	more	**pleo**morphic – Existing in more than one form.
		pleocytosis – Having more than the normal number of cells in cerebrospinal fluid.
pluri-	more	**pluri**glandular – Pertaining to several glands.
		pluripotency – Ability to develop in one of several ways or to affect several organs or tissues.
polio-	gray	**polio**clastic – Destruction of the gray matter of the nervous system.
		polioencephalitis – A disease of the gray matter in the brain.
poly-	many; much	**poly**chromatic – Having many colors.
		polyphagous – Eating many types of food.
post-	after; behind	**post**partum – Occurring after birth.
		postmortem – Occurring after death.
pre-	before	**pre**natal – Happening before birth.
		preterm – Happening before completion of the full term.
primi-	first	**primi**para – A woman who is pregnant for the first time.
		primitive – Pertaining to the first or early times.
pro-	before; forward	**pro**hibit – To stop before something happens.
		progression – To move forward.
quadri-	four	**quadri**ceps – A muscle with four heads.
		quadrigeminal – To have four parts.

MEDICAL PREFIX	MEANING	EXAMPLES
quasi-	as though	**quasi**dominance – Mimicking of dominance in inheritance caused by mating a carrier of a recessive gene with an individual homozygous for the gene.
rachi-	spine	**rachi**odynia – Pain of the spine.
		rachicentesis – A lumbar puncture.
re-	backwards; again	**re**traction – To draw back.
		repeat – To do again.
retro-	backward; behind	**retro**grade – To go backwards.
		retroflex – To bend backwards.
rhytid-	wrinkle	**rhytid** – A wrinkle in the skin.
		rhytidectomy – Surgical excision of skin to remove wrinkles.
sacchar-	sugar	**sacchar**ide – Among a group of carbohydrates, including the sugars.
		saccharin – Crystalline compound several hundred times sweeter than sucrose.
sangui-	blood	**sangui**facient – Pertaining to the formation of red blood cells.
		sanguinopurulent – Containing both blood and pus.
semi-	half	**semi**circle – Half of a circle.
		semicoma – A coma in which the patient can be aroused.
sub-	under, beneath; below; inferior	**sub**cutaneous – Under the skin.
		sublingual – Beneath the tongue.
sudo-	pertaining to sweat	**sudo**motor – To stimulate the sweat glands.
suf-	under; beneath; below; inferior	**suf**focation – Asphyxiation as by stoppage of respiration.
sup-	under, beneath; below; inferior	**sup**pression – To hold back or stop.
		suppository – A medication that is inserted through lower openings such as the anus.

MEDICAL PREFIX	MEANING	EXAMPLES
super-	above; beyond; in excess	**super**motility – More motility than normal.
		supernutrition – An excess of nutrition.
supra-	above; over	**supra**spinal – Above the spine.
		supracostal – Above the ribs.
sym-	with; together	**sym**pathomimetic – To mimic the effects caused by stimulation of the sympathetic nervous system.
		symphysis – To grow together.
syn-	with; together	**syn**desis – To bind together.
		syndrome – A set of symptoms that together characterize a disease. They "run their course together."
tachy-	swift; rapid; fast	**tachy**cardia – A rapid heart rate.
		tachyphagia – To eat rapidly.
taenia-	pertaining to tapeworms	**taenia**cide – Destroys tapeworms.
		taeniafuge – Expels tapeworms.
tele-	distance	**tele**kinesis – The movement of an object without contact.
		teletherapy – Treatment in which the agent does not contact the body.
ter-	thrice	**ter**nary – Third; made of three chemicals.
		tertian – Recurring every third day.
thi-	sulfur	**thi**ol – Sulfhydryl; containing -SH group.
trans-	through; across	**trans**lucent – Allowing light to pass through.
		transfusion – The process of introducing whole blood into the bloodstream.

MEDICAL PREFIX	MEANING	EXAMPLES
tri-	three	**tri**cep – A muscle with three heads.
		tricuspid – Having three points or cusps.
ultra-	excess; beyond	**ultra**sound – Sounds greater than the limit of human hearing.
		ultrahigh – Extremely high.
uni-	one	**uni**lateral – Having one side.
		unicellular – Made up of a single cell.
vermi-	worm	**vermi**cular – Resembling a worm.
		vermiculation – To move like a worm.
vivi-	alive	ovo**vivi**parous – Eggs are hatched within the body of the parent (e.g. snakes).
zo(o)-	animal	**zoo**logy – The study of animals.
		zoodermic – Done using the skin of an animal.

Medical Word Roots

"Better to light a light than complain about the darkness."

– Confucius

ROOTS

MEDICAL WORD ROOTS

MEDICAL ROOTS	MEANING	EXAMPLES
abdomin(o)	referring or pertaining to the abdomen	**abdomino**hysterectomy – A surgical procedure in which an abdominal approach is used to remove the uterus.
		abdominopelvic cavity – The cavity that includes the abdominal and pelvic cavities and is surrounded by the same serrous membrane, the peritoneum.
acanth(o)	a spine or thorn	**acantho**cyte – An abnormal red blood cell that appears "thorny."
		acantha – A vertebral spinous process.
acar(o)	mite	**acaro**dermatitis – A skin inflammation that is caused by mites.
		acarology – The study of mites and ticks.
acet(o)	vinegar	**acet**ic – Pertaining to vinegar; sour
acetabul(o)	pertaining or relating to the hip socket, by describing it as a "vinegar cup"	**acetabul**um – The cup-shaped socket of the hip joint.
		acetabuloplasty – Surgical repair of the acetabulum.
acoust(o)	pertaining or relating to the perception of sound	**acoust**ogram – A graph of the curves of sound.
		external **acoust**ic meatus – The external passage to the middle ear.
acr(o)	extremity; top	**acro**megaly – Enlargement of the extremities of the body (fingers, nose, jaw) by excessive growth hormone.
		acromion – The part of the scapula bone that forms the highest part of the shoulder.
actin(o)	ray	**actino**dermatitis – Radiodermatitis.
		actinotherapy – Treatment with ultraviolet rays.
acu(o)	sharpness, often related to sight or sound	**acu**ity – Pertaining to clarity.
		acupuncture – A mechanism to relieve pain by inserting needles in specific areas of the body.
aden(o)	pertaining or referring to a gland	**adeno**carcinoma – Carcinoma that originated from cells of glands.
		adenopathy – An increase in the size of glands often referring to lymph nodes.

MEDICAL ROOTS	MEANING	EXAMPLES
adenoid(o)	similar to a gland	**adenoid**ectomy – Surgical excision of the adenoids, lymphoid tissue located in the pharynx.
		adenoiditis – Inflammation of the adenoids.
adip(o)	pertaining or referring to fat	**adipo**cyte – A fat cell.
		adipsuria – Fat in the urine.
adren(o)	pertaining or referring to the adrenal gland	**adren**alin – A name for epinephrine, a hormone secreted by cells of the medulla of the adrenal gland.
		adrenomegaly – An increase in size of an adrenal gland.
aer(o)	pertaining or referring to air	**aero**be – A microorganism that lives in oxygen exposed environments.
		aeropathy – A disease process related to a change in atmospheric pressure.
agglutin(o)	adhering to one another; clumping	**agglutin**ation – Clumping of cells (often bacteria) after exposure to immunity system agents.
		agglutinin – An antibody which causes its antigen to clump to one another.
albin(o)	white	**albin**uria – Having white or pale urine.
		albinism – Not having normal pigmentation in the body.
albumin(o)	pertaining or referring to a protein	**albumin** – A soluble protein.
		albuminocholia – Protein in the bile.
algesi(o)	perception of pain	an**algesi**a – Without pain.
		an**algesic** – An agent that relieves pain.
alveol(o)	sac	pulmonary **alveol**i – Small sacs at the ends of terminal bronchioles in which respiratory gas exchange occurs.
		dental **alveol**i – The cavities in which the teeth are rooted.
ambly(o)	dull	**ambly**aphia – Decreased sharpness of touch perception.
		amblyacousia – Decreased sharpness of hearing.

MEDICAL ROOTS	MEANING	EXAMPLES
ambul(o)	walk	**ambul**atory – The ability to walk; not bedridden.
		ambulance – A "walking hospital."
amni(o)	pertaining to the membrane surrounding the fetus (i.e. amnion)	**amnio**tic fluid – Fluid surrounding the fetus.
		amniocentesis – The surgical procedure of inserting a needle through the abdominal wall and uterus to obtain amniotic fluid for tests.
ampulla	dilation of a tubular structure	**ampulla** of vater – The dilation of the pancreatic and common bile ducts as they merge before entering the duodenum.
		ampulla membranaceae – Dilation at the end of each semicircular duct.
amyl(o)	starch	**amylo**id – A substance resembling starch that is deposited in several disease states.
		amylose – A carbohydrate (except glucose or saccharose).
an(o)	anus	**ano**sigmoidoscopy – A procedure in which an endoscope is advanced through the anus to examine the rectum and sigmoid colon.
		anovaginal – Associated with the anus and vagina.
andr(o)	male	**andro**gen – A substance that induces male characteristics (e.g. testosterone).
		androblastoma – A benign tumor of the testicles.
aneurysm(o)	a dilation of the wall of an artery, vein, or the heart	**aneurysm**ectomy – Surgical excision of the aneurysm.
		aneurysmoplasty – Surgical repair of the aneurysm.
angi(o)	vessel	**angio**plasty – Surgical repair of blood vessels.
		angiography – Radiologic evaluation of blood vessels after injection of IV contrast dye.
angina	"squeezing" pain, often associated with lack of oxygen to the heart	**angina** pectoris – Pain associated with lack of oxygen to the heart.
		intestinal **angina** – Spasmodic pain associated with lack of oxygen to the abdominal viscera.

MEDICAL ROOTS	MEANING	EXAMPLES
anis(o)	unequal; not similar	**aniso**coria – Having pupils that are different in size.
		anisopiesis – Having varying blood pressure in different parts of the body.
ankyl(o)	crooked; fixed	**ankylo**sis – Inability of a joint to move.
		ankylosing spondylitis – A disease resulting in a severe immobility of the spine.
anthrac(o)	coal	**anthraco**necrosis – Necrosis of tissue into a black mass.
		anthracosis – A condition due to coal dust deposition in the lungs.
anthrop(o)	man	**anthropo**logy – The study of man.
		anthropometer – An instrument that measures body dimensions.
antr(o)	cavity	**antr**itis – Inflammation of an antrum, often describing the maxillary sinus (antrum).
		antrotymanic – Relating to the tympanic antrum and tympanum (middle ear cavity).
aort(o)	aorta	**aort**algia – Pain in or near the aorta.
		aortopathy – A disease of the aorta.
append(o)	relating or pertaining to an appendix (appendage)	**append**ectomy – Surgical excision of the vermiform appendix.
appendic(o)	relating or pertaining to an appendix (appendage)	**appendic**olysis – Surgical separation of adhesions from the vermiform appendix.
aque(o)	water	**aque**duct – A canal or channel.
		aqueous – Watery.
arachn(o)	spider	**arachno**id – Similar to a spider web. The arachnoid is the membrane between the pia mater and dura mater; all three form the meninges, which surrounds the brain.
		arachnodactyly – Unusually long and thin fingers and toes.

MEDICAL ROOTS	MEANING	EXAMPLES
arch(e)	first; origin	patri**arch** – A man considered to be a father or founder.
		men**arch**e – The onset of menstruation.
areola	a small area	**areola** – The small circular area of different pigment that surrounds the nipple of the breast.
		Chaussier's **areola** – The inflamed area immediately around a cancerous pustule.
argyr(o)	silver	**argyr**ia – Silver poisoning.
		argyrophil – Able to bind silver.
arteri(o)	artery	**arterio**sclerosis – Hardening of the arteries.
		arteritis – Inflammation of one or more arteries.
arteriol(o)	arteriole; a small artery	**arteriolo**necrosis – Degeneration of arterioles.
		arteriolosclerosis – Hardening of arterioles.
arthr(o)	joint	**arthr**algia – Pain of one or more joints.
		arthritis – Inflammation of one or more joints.
articul(o)	joint	**articul**ation – A joint between two bones.
		articulate – Divided by joints.
astr(o)	star	**astro**cyte – A star-shaped cell of the central nervous system which has an ectodermal origin.
		astrocytoma – A tumor of astrocytes.
atel(o)	incomplete or imperfect	**atel**ectasis – Incomplete expansion of the lungs.
		atelocardiac – Abnormal development of the heart.
ather(o)	relating or pertaining to cholesterol and fatty plaques found within the inner surface of arteries	**athero**sclerosis – A type of arteriosclerosis involving atheroma formation in arteries.
		atheroma – An intraluminal arterial plaque composed of cholesterol and lipid material.

MEDICAL ROOTS	MEANING	EXAMPLES
atri(o)	chamber that provides entrance into another location (often atrium)	right **atri**um – Provides entrance into the right ventricle of the heart.
		atriomegaly – Irregular enlargement of an atrium.
audi(o)	hearing	**audio**logy – The science of hearing.
		auditory – Pertaining or related to the ear or the perception of sound.
aur(o)	ear	**aur**icle – The appendage of the ear.
		auriculotemporal – Pertaining or related to the region of the ear and temple.
aux(o)	increase	**aux**esis – The increase in size of an organism.
		auxilytic – To increase in destructive ability.
axi(o)	axis	ab**axi**al – Away from the axis of a structure or part.
axill(o)	armpit	**axill**ary – Pertaining or related to the armpit.
		axilla – The armpit.
axon(o)	the axis	**axon** – The appendage of a neuron through which nerve signals are sent.
		axonometer – A device that estimates the axis of a lens.
azot(o)	urea; nitrogen-based waste	**azot**uria – Excessive nitrogen waste in the urine.
		azotemea – Excessive nitrogen waste in the blood.
ba(o)	walk; stand	a**ba**sia – Inability to walk.
bacteri(o)	bacteria	**bacteri**cidal – Something that kills bacteria.
		bacteremia – Bacteria in the blood.
balan(o)	pertaining or referring to the glans penis	**balano**plasty – Surgical repair of the glans penis.
		balanitis – Inflammation of the glans penis.
ball(o)	throw	**ball**ismus – Jerking of the limbs.

MEDICAL ROOTS	MEANING	EXAMPLES
bar(o)	weight	**baro**trauma – Injury caused by a change in pressure.
		barometer – An instrument for determining weight or pressure of the atmosphere.
bi(o)	life	aero**bi**c – Living in the presence of molecular oxygen.
		biogenesis – The origin of life.
blast(o)	bud; early stages of growth	**blasto**cyte – A primary germ cell.
		blastotomy – Separation of cells during the early stages of human development.
blephar(o)	eyelid	**blepharo**tomy – Surgical incision of the eyelid.
		blepharitis – Inflammation of the eyelid.
bol(o)	throw; ball	em**bol**ism – Blocking of an artery by a clot or object brought via blood flow.
		bolus – A rounded mass of food or pharmaceutical preparation made ready to swallow.
brachi(o)	arm	**brachi**al – Pertaining to the arm.
		brachialgia – Pain in the arm.
brachy(o)	short	**brachy**phalangia – Abnormal shortness of the phalanges.
		brachygnathia – Abnormal shortness of the lower jaw.
brom(o)	stench; foul odor	**brom**hidrosis – Sweat that has a foul odor.
		bromomenorrhea – Menstruation that has an offensive odor.
bronch(o)	windpipe; bronchus	**bronch**itis – Inflammation of one or more bronchi.
		bronchial – Pertaining to or associated with one or more bronchi.
bronchiol(o)	bronchiole	**bronchiol**ectasis – Dilation of the bronchioles.
bry(o)	life	em**bry**o – In humans, the developing organism up to the eighth week.
bucc(o)	cheek	**bucc**a – The cheek.

MEDICAL ROOTS	MEANING	EXAMPLES
bulb(o)	bulb	**bulb**ospiral – In reference to certain cardiac muscle pertaining to the root of the aorta and having a spiral course.
burs(o)	fluid-filled sac	**burs**a – A fluid-filled sac.
		bursitis – Inflammation of a bursa.
butyr(o)	butter	**butyr**oid – Resembling butter.
calc(o)	stone-like; heel; calcium	**calc**aneus – The heel bone.
		calcification – Hardening of tissue due to calcium deposition.
calor(o)	heat	**calor**imeter – An instrument for measuring heat.
		calorie – A unit of heat.
campt(o)	bent	**campto**dactyly – Having a permanently bent finger.
		camptomelia – A bending of the limbs that is permanent.
cancr(o)	cancer	**cancr**oid – Resembling cancer.
capit(a)	head	de**capit**ate – To cut off the head.
		capitate – Head-shaped.
carcin(o)	cancer	**carcino**gen – A substance that causes cancer.
		carcinoma – A cancerous tumor.
cardi(o)	heart	**cardio**megaly – Abnormal enlargement of the heart.
		cardiology – Study of the heart.
cari(o)	putrescence	**cari**es – Decay of bone or teeth.
		cariogenesis – The development of bone or tooth decay.
carp(o)	wrist	**carp**us – The wrist.
		carpectomy – Excision of a wrist bone.

MEDICAL ROOTS	MEANING	EXAMPLES
caud(o)	tail	**caud**ad – Toward the cauda (tail). In the human, this corresponds with the coccyx bone at the distal inferior end of the vertebral column.
		caudate – Having a tail.
caus(o)	burning	**caus**tic – The ability to burn; destroying living tissue.
		causalgia – Burning pain.
cauter(o)	burn	**cauter**y – An instrument that destroys tissue by burning.
		cauterize – To burn with a cautery.
cec(o)	cecum; blind	**cec**al – pertaining or associated with a blind passage; the cecum.
		cecitis – Inflammation of the cecum.
celi(o)	abdomen	**celio**ma – A tumor of the abdomen.
		celiac – Associated with the abdomen.
cell(o)	room; cell	**cell**ular – Pertaining to or made of cells; consisting of small compartments.
cement(o)	cement	**cement**um – The bone-like covering of the root of the tooth.
cephal(o)	head	**cephalo**pod – A mollusk belonging to the class cephalopoda, which are defined by having tentacles attached to a large head.
		cephalomegaly – Enlargement of the head.
cer(o)	wax	**cer**oplasty – Making anatomical models in wax.
		cerumen – Earwax.
cerc(o)	tail	**cerc**aria – The larval form of a trematode worm whose body is terminated by a tail-like appendage.
		Hetero**cerc**al – In animals, a vertebral column continued into the upper lobe of the tail.

MEDICAL ROOTS	MEANING	EXAMPLES
cerebell(o)	cerebellum	**cerebell**ar – Associated with or pertaining to the cerebellum.
		cerebellitis – Inflammation of the cerebellum.
cerebr(o)	brain	**cerebr**um – The main portion of the brain.
		cerebrospinal – Pertaining to the brain and spinal cord.
cervic(o)	neck; cervix (neck of the uterus)	**cervico**thoracic – Pertaining to the neck and thorax.
		cervicitis – Inflammation of the cervix of the uterus.
chem(o)	chemical	**chemo**therapy – Treatment of disease through the use of chemicals.
		chemosurgery – Use of chemicals to destroy diseased tissue.
chol(e)	bile	**chol**agogue – A substance that causes bladder contraction in order to promote bile flow.
		cholelithiasis – Formation of stones in the biliary system.
cholangi(o)	Relating to the bile duct	**cholangio**graphy – The use of radiography to examine the bile ducts.
		cholangiectasis – Dilation of a bile duct.
cholecyst(o)	gallbladder	**cholecyst**itis – Inflammation of the gallbladder.
		cholecystectomy – Surgical excision of the gallbladder.
choledoch(o)	common bile duct	**choledoch**al – Pertaining to the common bile duct.
		choledochitis – Inflammation of the common bile duct.
chondr(o)	cartilage	**chondro**blast – A cell that produces cartilage that is in the early stages of growth.
		chondropathy – Disease of the cartilage.
chor(o)	membrane	**chor**ion – The outer membrane surrounding the embryo in reptiles, birds, and mammals.
		choroid – A membrane that coats the eye that is found between the sclera and the retina.
chord(o)	cord	**chord**ate – Having a notochord.
		chorditis – Inflammation of a vocal or spermatic cord.

MEDICAL ROOTS	MEANING	EXAMPLES
chore(o)	dance	**chore**a – A condition characterized by rapid, jerky, involuntary movements.
		choreography – A sequence of movements, as in dance.
chrom(o)	color	a**chrom**asia – Hypopigmentation; lack of staining power in a cell or tissue.
		chromoblast – Embryonic cell that develops into a pigment cell.
chromat(o)	color	poly**chromat**ic – Having many colors.
		chromaturia – Abnormal urine color.
chron(o)	time	ana**chron**ism – Not in the correct historical time; out of chronological order.
		chronic – Constant; existing for a long time.
chrys(o)	gold	**chryso**derma – A permanent change in pigmentation of the skin due to gold deposits.
		chrysotherapy – Treatment with gold salts.
chyl(i)	juice	**chyl**e – The milky fluid taken up by the lacteals from food in the instestine.
		chyliform – Resembling chyle.
cine(o)	movement	**cine**matography – The making of a motion picture or film.
		cineradiography – Making a motion picture of successive x-rays.
cirs(o)	varix (varicose vessels)	**cirs**oid – Resembling a varix (a large twisting blood or lymphatic vessel).
cleid(o)	clavicle	**cleid**ocranial – Pertaining to the clavicle and the head.
clin(o)	incline; bend; bed	**clin**ic – A place where instruction is given at the bedside.
		clinoid – Shaped like a bed.
coccyg(o)	coccyx	**coccyg**eal – Pertaining to or associated with the coccyx.
		coccygectomy – Surgical excision of the coccyx.

MEDICAL ROOTS	MEANING	EXAMPLES
col(o)	large intestine	**col**itis – Inflammation of the colon.
		colic – Abdominal pain.
colp(o)	vagina	**colp**algia – Pain in the vagina.
		colpohyperplasia – Excessive thickening of the wall of the vagina.
condyl(o)	rounded projection	**condyl**e – A rounded projection on the bone.
		condyloma – A growth on the skin.
coni(o)	dust	**coni**osis – A disease caused by dust.
		pneumo**coni**osis – A lung disease caused by the inhalation of dust.
copr(o)	feces	**copro**phobia – Fear of feces.
		coprostasis – Fecal impactation in the intestine.
cor(o)	pupil; with; together	**cor**nea – The transparent part of the eye.
		corectasis – Dilation of the pupil.
		correlate – Ability to associate one phenomena with another.
coron(o)	associated with or pertaining to the coronary arteries; crown-shaped	**coron**ary – Encircling like a crown; associated with the heart.
		coronoid – Crown-shaped.
corp(o)	body	**corp**se – A dead body.
cortic(o)	bark; outer layer; cortex	**cortico**trophin – A hormone that stimulates the adrenal cortex.
		corticolous – Living on bark.
cost(o)	rib	**cost**algia – Pain in the ribs.
		inter**cost**al – Between the ribs.

MEDICAL WORD ROOTS

MEDICAL ROOTS	MEANING	EXAMPLES
crani(o)	skull	**cranio**tomy – Surgery in which the skull is opened.
		craniomalacia – Unusual softening of the skull.
creat(o)	meat	**creat**ine – Amino acid which occurs mostly in muscle tissue and is important in storing high-energy phosphate.
cret(o)	distinguish; separate; growth	ac**cret**ion – Growth by accumulation.
		dis**cret**e – Made up of separate parts.
crur(o)	shin, leg	**crur**al – Pertaining to or resembling a lower limb.
		talo**crur**al – Pertaining to the talus and the leg bones.
cry(o)	cold	**cryo**anesthesia – Anesthesia caused by chilling to a near freezing temperature.
		cryogenic – Very low temperatures.
crypt(o)	hide	**crypto**genic – Of an obscure origin.
		cryptomenorrhea – Menstrual systems without external bleeding.
cutane(o)	skin	sub**cutaneo**us – Under the skin.
		per**cutaneo**us – Given through or by way of the skin.
cyan(o)	blue	**cyano**bacteria – Blue-green algae.
		cyanopsia – A problem with the eye that causes things to appear blue.
cycl(o)	circle; ciliary body of the eye	**cyclo**ne – A rotating windstorm; tornado.
		cyclotomy – Surgical incision of the ciliary muscle.
cymb(o)	boat	**cymb**ocephaly – Abnormal length and narrowness of the skull.
cyn(o)	dog	**cyn**ophobia – Fear of dogs.
cyst(o)	bladder	**cyst**itis – Inflammation of the bladder.
		cystalgia – Pain in the bladder.

MEDICAL ROOTS	MEANING	EXAMPLES
cyt(o)	cell	**cyto**kinesis – Final stage of cell division when the cytoplasm splits.
		cytology – The study of cells.
dacry(o)	tear; lacrimal gland of the eye	**dacry**ops – An excess of tears.
		dacryoadenalgia – Pain of the lacrimal gland.
dactyl(o)	digit	campto**dactyl**y – Having a permanently bent finger.
		hexa**dactyl**y – Having six fingers or toes on a hand or foot.
dendr(o)	tree; branching	**dendro**logy – The study of trees.
		dendrite – One of the branches of a nerve cell that receives impulses.
dent(o)	tooth	**dent**algia – A toothache.
		dentist – A person who works on teeth.
derm(o)	skin	**derm**atology – A branch of medicine that deals with the skin.
		erythro**derm**a – An abnormal redness of the skin.
desm(o)	ligament	**desmo**plasia – Formation of a ligament.
		desmotomy – Surgical incision of a ligament.
dextr(o)	right (side)	ambi**dextro**us – Can use either hand well.
		dextrorotatory – Turning toward the right side.
dicty(o)	nest	**dicty**otene – Stage in which the primary oocyte spends from late fetal life until discharged from ovary.
didym(o)	twin; testis	**didymo**us – Existing in pairs or twins.
		epi**didym**is – The structure where sperm are stored.
dipl(o)	double	**diplo**pia – Seeing two of a single object.
		diploid – Having two sets of chromosomes.

MEDICAL ROOTS	MEANING	EXAMPLES
dips(o)	thirst	**dipso**gen – Something that induces thirst.
		dipsosis – Excessive thirst.
disc(o)	disk	**disc**ogenic – Caused by derangement of an intervertebral disk.
		discoplacenta – Discoid placenta.
dolor(o)	pain	**dolor**imeter – An instrument for measuring pain.
		dolorology – The study of pain.
dors(o)	back	**dorso**ventral – Associated with or pertaining to the back and belly.
		dorsiflexion – Bending towards the back.
drom(o)	course	**dromo**graph – A instrument for recording the rate at which blood flows through the body.
		syn**drom**e – A set of symptoms that together characterize a disease; they "run their course together."
duct(o)	lead; tube; duct	ab**duct** – Lead away from the medial plane.
		ovi**duct** – A duct that allows the ova or egg to the leave from the ovary and pass to the uterus.
duoden(o)	duodenum	**duoden**itis – Inflammation of the duodenum.
		duodenum – The first portion of the small intestine.
dur(o)	hard	in**dur**ation – Hardening; In medicine, an area of the body that has hardened.
		dura mater – The tough, outermost membrane of the brain.
dynam(o)	power	**dynam**ic – Pertaining to or associated with force.
		cardio**dynam**ics – The study of the forces associated with pumping blood in the heart.
ech(o)	have; hold	syn**ech**ia – An adhesion, as of the iris to the cornea or lens.
echin(o)	hedgehog	**echin**ocyte – A spiky cell.

MEDICAL ROOTS	MEANING	EXAMPLES
ectr(o)	miscarriage; congenital absence	**ectro**dactyly – Absence of a finger or toe.
		ectrogeny – The absence or defect of a part.
elast(o)	elasticity	**elast**oma – Local tumorlike excess of elastic tissue fibers.
		elastometry – Measurement of elasticity.
encephal(o)	brain	**encephalo**pathy – Any pathological condition affecting the brain.
		encephalitis – Inflammation of the brain.
enter(o)	intestine	**entero**centesis – Surgical puncture of the intestine.
		enteroparesis – Relaxation of the intestine, resulting in dilation.
entom(o)	insect	**entom**ology – Study of insects.
		entomophthorales – An order of fungi that typically parasitically infects insects.
eosin(o)	red; rosy	**eosino**penia – A low number of eosinophils in the blood.
		eosinophil – A white blood cell that stains with red dye.
epipl(o)	omentum	**epipl**oic – Pertaining to the omentum.
episi(o)	pubic region	**episi**ostenosis – Narrowing of the vulvar orifice.
		episiotomy – An incision made into the perineum and vagina to prevent tearing during delivery.
erg(o)	work	**ergo**nomics – The study of humans in the workplace.
		ex**ergo**nic – The release of energy.
erot(o)	relating to or associated with sexual desire	**eroto**phobia – Fear of sexual desire.
		erotism – One's sexual desire.
erythr(o)	red	**erythro**cyte – Red blood cell.

MEDICAL WORD ROOTS

MEDICAL ROOTS	MEANING	EXAMPLES
esthe(s)	feeling; sensation	an**esthesia** – The loss of sensation.
		hyp**esthesia** – A decrease in sensation.
estr(o)	female	**estro**gen – A female hormone.
eti(o)	cause	**etio**logy – Study of the cause of disease.
faci(o)	face	**facio**plasty – Plastic surgery of the face.
		facioplegia – Paralysis of the face.
fasci(o)	band	**fasci**a – A sheet or band of fibrous tissue.
		fasciotomy – Surgical incision of a fascia.
febr(o)	fever	a**febr**ile – Without fever.
		febricity – Having a fever.
fec(o)	feces	**fec**ulent – Pertaining to or associated with feces.
		fecalith – A hard mass of feces.
femor(o)	femur	**femor**ocele – Femoral hernia.
ferr(o)	iron	**ferr**odoxin – Nonheme iron-containing protein.
		ferroprotein – Protein combined with an iron-containing radical.
fet(o)	fetus	**feto**metry – Measurement of the fetus.
		fetology – A branch of medicine dealing with the fetus.
fibr(o)	fiber	**fibro**ma – A tumor composed of mainly fibrous tissue.
		fibrochondritis – Inflammation of fibrocartilage.
flagell(o)	whip	**flagell**a – Long, whiplike appendages attached to the surface of a cell that propel the organism.
		flagellation – Whipping one's self for pleasure; the formation of flagella on an organism.

MEDICAL ROOTS	MEANING	EXAMPLES
flect(o)	bend	de**flect**ion – Deviation from a straight line.
		in**flect**ion – The act or state of bending inward.
flex(o)	bend	re**flex** – Action or movement brought on by the automatic response of the nervous system.
		flexion – The act or condition of bending.
flu(x)	flow	**flu**id – A liquid or gas.
		de**flux**ion – Sudden disappearance; copious discharge; falling out (e.g. hair).
follicul(o)	follicle	**follicul**ar – Related to one or more follicles.
		folliculitis – Inflammation of a follicle.
for(o)	bore	imper**for**ate – Abnormally closed.
		foramen – Naturally occuring opening or passage (e.g. into bone).
fract(o)	break	**fract**al – Curve or geometric figure, each part of which has the same statistical character as the whole.
		fracture – Breaking of a part (e.g. bone).
fug(i)	flee	**fug**ue – State of altered consciousness in which the individual wanders aimlessly, not guided by his normal personality and which is not remembered afterwards.
		centri**fug**ation – Process of separating heavy particles from lighter particles using centrifugal force.
funct(o)	perform	de**funct** – Dead; no longer existing or able to function.
fund(i)	pour	in**fund**ibulum – Funnel shaped structure.
		fundiform – Shaped like a loop or sling.
furc(o)	fork	**furc**ula – A forked bone, the wishbone or furculum.
		furcation – To branch like a fork.

MEDICAL WORD ROOTS

MEDICAL ROOTS	MEANING	EXAMPLES
fus(o)	flow; spindle	dif**fus**e – To pass through or spread widely throughout a tissue or structure.
		fusible – Able to be melted.
galact(o)	milk	**galacto**phore – Milk duct.
		galactorrhea – Excessive flow of milk.
gamet(o)	marriage; reproduction	**gamet**e – One of two haploid reproductive cells, male or female; malarial parasite in its sexual form.
		gametogenesis – Development of the male and female sex cells.
gangli(o)	ganglion; swelling; knot	**ganglio**nitis – Inflammation of a ganglion.
		ganglionectomy – Surgical excision of a ganglion.
gastr(o)	stomach	**gastro**pathy – A disease of the stomach.
		gastrin – A hormone that stimulates secretion of juices in the stomach.
gelat(o)	freeze; congeal	**gelat**ion – To solidify by cooling.
gen(i)	chin	**geni**culum – Anatomical nomenclature for a sharp bend in a small structure or organ.
gen(o)	begin; originate; produce	carcino**gen**ic – A cancer producing agent.
		generation – Reproduction.
genit(o)	referring to birth	**genit**alia – The reproductive organs, more often referring to those that are external.
		genitourinary – Pertaining to the genital and urinary systems.
ger(o)	old age	**ger**iatrics – Medicine that deals with the elderly.
		gerodontics – Dentistry that deals with the elderly.
germ(o)	bud; seed; bacteria	**germ**icide – An agent that kills bacteria.
		germination – Beginning to grow.
gest(o)	bear; carry	in**gest**ant – Substance that is taken into the body by mouth or through the digestive system.

MEDICAL ROOTS	MEANING	EXAMPLES
gingiv(o)	gum	**gingiv**itis – Inflammation of the gums.
		gingiva – The gum.
gland(o)	acorn	**gland**ular – Pertaining or similar to a gland.
glauc(o)	glaucoma	**glauco**matous – Pertaining to or associated with glaucoma.
gli(o)	glue	neuro**gli**a – A type of cells in the brain and spinal cord that provide support for neurons.
		glioma – A tumor composed of neuroglia.
glomerul(o)	little ball	**glomerul**us – A small cluster (e.g. blood vessels or nerve fibers).
gloss(o)	tongue	**gloss**ectomy – Surgical excision of all or a portion of the tongue.
		glossotrichia – A hairy tongue.
glott(o)	tongue; language	**glott**is – Vocal apparatus of the larnyx.
		glottography – Record of the movements of the vocal cords.
gluc(o)	pertaining to or associated with glucose	**gluco**neogenesis – The production of glucose.
		glucophore – An amino derivative of glucose.
glutin(o)	glue	ag**glutin**ant – Causes adhesive union; substance that holds parts together during healing.
		glutinous – Adhesive.
glyc(o)	sugar	**glyco**lysis – The breakdown of glucose.
		hyper**glyc**emia – Elevated blood sugar level.
gnath(o)	jaw	**gnatho**schisis – Cleft jaw.
		a**gnath**a – A class of jawless chordates.
gno(s)	knowledge; know	dia**gnos**is – Knowing the cause of a problem or situation.
		pro**gno**stic – Predicting the outcome.

MEDICAL WORD ROOTS

MEDICAL ROOTS	MEANING	EXAMPLES
gon(o)	offspring; genitalia; knee	**gon**ad – Gamete producing gland (e.g. ovary or testis).
		gonarthritis – Inflammation of the knee.
gonad(o)	reproductive glands	**gonado**toxic – Having a harmful effect of the gonads.
		gonadectomy – Surgical removal of an ovary or testis.
goni(o)	angle	**gonio**meter – An instrument used to measure angles.
		gonioscope – An instrument for examining the angular motion of the eye.
granul(o)	granular; grainy	**granulo**cytopenia – A decrease in granular leukocytes.
		granuloma – A tumor composed of granular tissue.
gravid(o)	pregnancy	**gravid**a – A pregnant woman.
		gravidocardiac – Heart disease during pregnancy.
gust(o)	taste	**gust**atory – Pertaining to or associated with taste.
		gustin – A polypeptide present in saliva.
gymn(o)	naked	**gymn**osperm – Seed that is unprotected by ovary or fruit.
gynec(o)	woman	**gyneco**logy – A branch of medicine dealing with women.
		gynephobia – Fear of women.
gyr(o)	ring; circle	**gyr**ospasm – Spasm in which the head rotates around the neck.
		gyrate – Revolve around a fixed point.
hal(o)	breath	ex**hal**e – To breathe out.
		halitosis – Bad breath.
hamart(o)	fault	**hamart**oma – Benign tumor-like nodule in which cells normally present are disorderly and out of proportion.
hapt(o)	touch	**hapt**ics – Study of the sense of touch.

MEDICAL ROOTS	MEANING	EXAMPLES
hel(o)	nail; callus	**hel**oma – A corn.
helc(o)	sore; ulcer	kerato**helc**osis – Ulcer of the cornea.
helic(o)	coil	**helic**opod – A dragging gait.
		helical – Spiral.
hem(o)	blood	**hem**atemesis – Vomiting blood.
		hemoglobin – A protein found in red blood cells.
hemangi(o)	blood vessel	**hemangio**ma – A tumor made up of blood vessels.
		hemangioblast – A developing cell that gives rise to blood vessels.
hepat(o)	liver	**hepat**itis – Inflammation of the liver.
		hepatomegaly – Enlargement of the liver.
hered(i)	heir	**hered**itary – Genetically passed from parent to child.
herni(o)	hernia; rupture	**herni**ated – To stick out abnormally.
		hernioplasty – Surgery to repair a hernia.
herpet(o)	crawl; snake	**herpet**ology – Study of snakes.
heter(o)	other; different	**hetero**geneous – Made of different substances; not alike.
		heterocrine – Secreting more than one substance or matter.
hex(o)	have; be	cac**hex**ia – State of ill health and malnutrition.
hidr(o)	sweat	**hidro**tic – Sweating an abnormal amount.
		dys**hidro**sis – A disorder of the sweat glands.
hipp(o)	horse	**hipp**ocampus – Curved elevation in the floor of the inferior horn of the lateral ventricle.
		hippodrome – Arena set apart for horse and chariot races.

MEDICAL WORD ROOTS

MEDICAL ROOTS	MEANING	EXAMPLES
hist(o)	tissue	**histo**kinesis – Movement of tissues in the body.
		histology – The study of tissues in the body.
hod(o)	path	**hod**oneuromere – Segment of the embryonic trunk.
home(o)	like; resembling; constant	**homeo**stasis – Staying in a constant state; equilibrium.
		homeothermy – The maintaining of constant body temperature.
horm(o)	impulse	**horm**one – A chemical impulse sent to affect certain cells or organs.
hyal(o)	glass-like	**hyal**ine – Glassy or translucent.
		hyaloplasm – A glass-like fluid found in the cell.
hydr(o)	water	**hydr**ation – To combine or supply with water.
		hydrophobic – Not absorbing water.
hymen(o)	membrane	**hymen** – A membrane that covers part of the entrance to the vagina.
		hymenology – The study of the membranes of the body.
hypn(o)	sleep	**hypno**sis – To put someone in a sleep-like state.
		hypnalgia – Pain during sleep.
hyps(o)	height	**hyps**okinesis – A swaying or falling when in erect posture.
hyster(o)	uterus; womb	**hyster**ectomy – Surgical excision of the uterus.
		hysteropathy – A disease of the uterus.
iatr(o)	physician	ped**iatr**ician – A physician who treats children.
		iatrogenic – Caused by the medical treatment of a physician.
ichthy(o)	fish	**ichthyo**sis – A disorder of the skin that causes scaliness, like fish skin.
		ichthyic – Pertaining to or like fish.

MEDICAL ROOTS	MEANING	EXAMPLES
icter(o)	jaundice	**ictero**genic – Causing jaundice.
		icterohepatitis – Inflammation or the liver marked by jaundice.
idi(o)	distinct; separate; peculiar; self	**idio**pathic – Having no known cause.
		idiomorphic – Having a distinct form.
igni(o)	fire	**igni**te – To light on fire.
		ignipuncture – Puncture of the body using hot instruments for therapeutic purposes.
ile(o)	ileum; the longest portion of the intestine	**ile**ectomy – Surgical excision of the ileum.
		ileitis – Inflammation of the ileum.
ili(o)	pertaining or referring to the ilium or hip bone	**ili**ac – Referring to the hip bone.
		iliocostal – Connecting or referring to the hip bone and ribs.
immun(o)	resistance; protection	**immun**ization – To make immune or resistant to, particularly by innoculation.
		immunosuppressant – To prevent an immune response.
in(o)	fiber	**in**otropic – Affecting the force of muscular contractions.
insul(o)	island	**insul**in – A hormone that is produced by the islets of Langerhans.
		insulate – To surround or make an island of.
irid(o)	iris	**irido**plegia – Paralysis of the sphincter of the iris.
		iridocyclitis – Inflammation of the iris and ciliary body.
isch(o)	suppress	**isch**emia – A decrease in blood supply.
		ischuria – A decrease in urine flow.
ischi(o)	hip; haunch; ischium	**ischio**dynia – Pain in the ischium.
		ischiorectal – Pertaining to the ischium and rectum.

MEDICAL WORD ROOTS

MEDICAL ROOTS	MEANING	EXAMPLES
jact(i)	throw	**jact**itation – Restless back and forth or side to side movement during acute illness.
jejun(o)	empty; jejunum	gastro**jejuno**stomy – Surgery to make a new passage between the stomach and jejunum.
		jejunotomy – Surgical incision of the jejunum.
jug(u)	yoke; neck	con**jug**ate – Paired; working together.
		jugular – Of or pertaining to the neck or throat.
junct(o)	join	con**junct**iva – Membrane covering the eyeball.
kal(i)	potassium	**kali**uresis – Potassium in the urine.
		hyper**kal**emia – An elevated amount of potassium in the blood.
kary(o)	nucleus	**karyo**rrhexis – Rupture of the cell nucleus.
		karyokinesis – Division of the cell nucleus.
kerat(o)	horn-like; cornea	**kerat**in – A protein that makes up horny tissues of the body.
		keratocentesis – Puncture of the cornea.
kine(o)	movement	hyper**kine**sia – Excessive movement.
		kinesitherapy – The treatment of disease through massage and exercise.
klept(o)	to steal	**klept**omania – Compulsive stealing of objects with no personal or monetary value.
koil(o)	hollow	**koilo**cyte – A hollow cell.
		koilonychia – A condition in which the fingernails are concave and have raised edges.
labi(o)	lip	**labio**mental – Pertaining to the lip and chin.
		labiochorea – A spasm of the lips that interferes during speech.
lacrim(o)	tears; tear duct	**lacrim**ator – Something that induces the flow of tears.
		lacrimotomy – Surgical incision of the lacrimal duct or sac.

MEDICAL ROOTS	MEANING	EXAMPLES
lact(o)	milk	**lacto**bacillus – A bacteria found in milk.
		lactogen – Something that enhances milk production.
lal(o)	talk	glosso**lal**ia – Nosense talk that mirrors coherent speech.
		lallation – Infantile speech.
lamin(o)	thin layer or sheet; posterior arch of vertebra	**lamin**ated – Arranged in layers.
		laminectomy – Surgical excision of the posterior arch of a vertebra.
lapar(o)	flank; loin; abdomen	**laparo**tomy – Surgical incision of the abdomen.
		laparoscopy – The use of a laparoscope to examine the inside of the abdomen.
laryng(o)	larynx	**laryngo**plegia – Paralysis of the larynx.
		laryngostenosis – A narrowing of the larynx.
lat(o)	carry	corre**lat**e – Ability to associate one phenomena with another.
		trans**lat**e – Convert; process of codons in mRNA being converted to the sequence of amino acids constituting a polypeptide chain.
later(o)	to the side	ventro**later**al – Pertaining to the front and side.
		lateroversion – A turning to one side.
lax(a)	loosen; widen	**laxa**tive – Something that widens the intestinal tract or loosens stool.
		re**lax** – To make less tense or loosen the muscles.
lecith(o)	yolk	iso**lecith**al – Yolk evenly distributed throughout the cytoplasm as in mammalian eggs.
		lecithal – Having yolk.
lei(o)	smooth	**leio**dermia – Smooth skin.
		leiomyoma – A tumor that is made up of smooth muscle.

MEDICAL WORD ROOTS

MEDICAL ROOTS	MEANING	EXAMPLES
lept(o)	thin; slender; delicate	**lepto**cephalus – Having an abnormally narrow skull.
		leptotene – A stage of cell division which occurs during prophase of meiosis I in which the chromosomes are threadlike.
leuk(o)	white	**leuko**cyte – White blood cell.
		leukoplakia – White patches on the mucous membrane.
lev(o)	left	**lev**orotatory – Turning the plane of polarization of polarized light to the left.
lien(o)	spleen	gastro**lien**al – Pertaining to the stomach and the spleen.
		lienomalacia – Softening of the spleen.
lig(o)	tie; bind	**lig**ase – An enzyme that joins together molecules.
		ligament – Tissue that connects bones or cartilage.
lingu(o)	tongue	bi**lingu**al – Speaking two languages.
		sub**lingu**al – Beneath the tongue.
lip(o)	fat	**lipo**lysis – The breakdown of fat.
		lipoid – To resemble fat.
lith(o)	stone	nephro**litho**tripsy – Removal of kidney stones.
		lithuresis – Small stones in the urine.
lob(o)	lobe	**lob**ectomy – Surgical excision of a lobe.
		lobation – Forming of lobes.
log(o)	speak; speech	**log**apathy – A speech disorder.
		logoplegia – Paralysis of speech organs.
loph(o)	tuft	**loph**otrichous – Having two or more flagella at one end.
lord(o)	bent; curved	**lord**osis – A curving of the spine.

MEDICAL ROOTS	MEANING	EXAMPLES
luc(o)	light; shine; transparent	trans**luc**ent – Allowing light to pass through.
		lucent – Clear; shining.
lumb(o)	loin; lower back	**lumbo**sacral – Associated with or pertaining to the loins and sacrum.
		lumbar – Associated with or pertaining to the lower back.
lumin(o)	light; cavity inside a tubular structure	**lumin**escence – To give off light without heat.
		luminal – Associated with or pertaining to a cavity in a tubular organ.
lute(o)	yellow	**lute**in – A yellow pigment.
		luteoma – A yellow tumor found in the ovary.
lymph(o)	lymph; water	**lymph**edema – Swelling caused by build up of lymph.
		lymphostasis – To stop the flow of lymph.
lymphaden(o)	lymph nodes	**lymphaden**ocele – Cyst on the lymph node.
		lymphadenitis – Inflammation of a lymph node.
lymphangi(o)	lymph vessel	**lymphangi**ectasis – Dilation of a lymph vessel.
		lymphangioma – A tumor made up of forming lymph spaces and channels.
lys(o)	breakdown; split; dissolution	lipo**lys**is – The breakdown of fat.
		hydro**lys**is – The splitting of water molecules.
mamm(o)	breast	**mammo**gram – An x-ray of the breast.
		sub**mamm**ary – Below the breast.
mandibul(o)	mandible	**mandibul**a – The mandible.
		mandibular – Associated with or pertaining to the mandible.
man(i)	hand	**man**ipulation – Skillful use of the hands.

MEDICAL WORD ROOTS

MEDICAL ROOTS	MEANING	EXAMPLES
mast(o)	breast	hyper**mast**ia – Enlargement of the breasts.
		mastectomy – Surgical removal of the breast.
maxill(o)	upper jaw	**maxillo**mandibular – Associated with or pertaining to the upper and lower jaws.
		sub**maxill**ary – Beneath the jaw.
meat(o)	course; passage	**meat**us – An opening or passage.
		meatotomy – Surgical incision of the urinary passage.
mechan(o)	machine	**mechan**oreceptor – A receptor that responds to mechanical pressures or distortions.
mel(o)	limb; cheek	sym**mel**ia – A developmental anomaly characterized by a fusion of the lower limbs.
		meloplasty – Plastic sugery of the cheek.
melan(o)	black; melanin	**melano**cyte – A cell which produces melanin or pigment.
		melanonychia – Blackening of the nails.
men(o)	menstruation	hypo**meno**rrhea – A decreased menstrual flow.
		menarche – The onset of menstruation.
mening(o)	meninges; membrane	**meningo**malacia – Softening of a membrane.
		meningitis – Inflammation of the meninges.
ment(o)	mind; chin	**mento**labial – Associated with or pertaining to the chin and lip.
		mentoplasty – Plastic surgery on the chin.
mer(o)	thigh	**mer**algia – Pain of the thigh.
mes(o)	middle	**meso**derm – The middle germ layer of a forming embryo.
		mesiad – Toward the middle.

MEDICAL ROOTS	MEANING	EXAMPLES
metr(o)	uterus; womb	**metro**plasty – Plastic surgery on the uterus.
		metrorrhea – An abnormal discharge from the uterus.
mi(o)	smaller; less	**mio**sis – Contraction of the pupil.
		miosphygmia – A condition in which there are fewer pulse beats than there are heart beats.
micr(o)	small	**micro**scopic – Too small to be seen with the unaided eye.
		microstomia – An unusually small mouth.
morph(o)	shape; form	**morpho**logy – The study of shape and form.
		zoo**morph**ic – Having the form of an animal.
mort(o)	fatal; death	**mort**al – Pertaining to death; deadly.
		im**mort**ality – Having a life that is unending.
muc(o)	mucus	**muc**inosis – Having an elevated amount of mucins in the skin.
		mucopurulent – Having both mucus and pus.
mut(a)	mutation; change	**muta**gen – A substance that induces genetic mutation.
		mutase – An enzyme that changes chemical groups by shifting them from one position to another.
my(o)	muscle	**myo**globin – A protein found in the muscle.
		myasthenia – Muscular weakness (e.g. myasthenia gravis).
myc(o)	fungus	dermato**myco**sis – A fungal infection of the skin.
		onycho**myco**sis – A fungal infection of the nails.
myel(o)	bone marrow; spinal cord	**myel**itis – Inflammation of the spinal cord.
		myeloma – A tumor that is made up of bone marrow cells.

MEDICAL WORD ROOTS

MEDICAL ROOTS	MEANING	EXAMPLES
myring(o)	membrane; eardrum	**myringo**plasty – Surgical repair of the eardrum.
		myringectomy – Surgical excision of the eardrum.
myx(o)	mucus	**myx**asthenia – A low secretion of mucus.
		myxadenitis – Inflammation of a mucous gland.
narc(o)	numb; stupor; sleep	**narco**lepsy – A disorder that causes uncontrolled episodes of deep sleep.
		narcosis – A sleep-like state.
nas(o)	nose	para**nas**al – Adjacent to the nose.
		nasopharynx – The part of the pharynx that is continuous with the nasal passages.
nat(i)	birth	neo**nat**al – Pertaining to a newborn child.
		natalitial – Associated with or pertaining to a birth or birthday.
natr(o)	salt; sodium	**natr**iuresis – Excretion of sodium in the urine.
		hyper**natr**emia – An elevated amount of sodium in the blood.
nebul(o)	cloud; fog; mist	**nebul**a – A cloudy spot on the cornea.
		nebulize – To make into a mist.
necr(o)	death; corpse	**necro**sis – The death of tissue.
		necrophobia – Fear of death or dead bodies.
nephr(o)	kidney	**nephro**lithotripsy – Removal of kidney stones.
		nephrology – The study of the kidneys.
neur(o)	nerve	**neur**ectopia – Abnormal placement of a nerve.
		neuralgia – Sharp pain along the course of a nerve.
neutr(o)	neutral; neither	**neutro**n – A particle that has no charge.
		neutrophil – A cell that can be stained by neutral dyes.

MEDICAL ROOTS	MEANING	EXAMPLES
nev(o)	mole	**nev**olipoma – Nevus with a large amount of fibrofatty tissue.
		nevus – Birthmark; congenital skin lesion; hamartoma consisting of a stable, circumscribed, malformation of the skin.
noci(a)	injure	**noci**ceptor – Receptor for pain.
noct(i)	night	**noct**uria – To urinate frequently during the night.
		noctambulism – Sleepwalking.
nod(o)	knot	**nod**osity – A node or having nodes.
nom(i)	law; custom	taxo**nom**y – The orderly classification of organisms into appropriate groupings.
norm(o)	usual; pattern	**normo**tensive – Having normal blood pressure.
		normocyte – An erythrocyte that is normal according to size, shape, and color.
nos(o)	disease	**nos**ocomial – Pertaining to or coming from a hospital (often referring to diseases transmitted in hospitals).
		nosology – Scientific classification of diseases.
nucle(o)	nucleus	**nucleo**plasm – The protoplasm found in the nucleus of a cell.
		nucleoprotein – Proteins found in the nucleus of a cell.
nutri(o)	nourish	mal**nutri**tion – Not having good nutrition.
		nutrient – A nourishing substance.
nyct(o)	night	**nyct**alopia – Night blindness.
		nyctophobia – Fear of darkness.
nymph(o)	bride	**nymph**otomy – Surgical excision of the nymphae (i.e. clitoris).
occip(o)	back of the head	**occip**ut – The back of the head.

MEDICAL ROOTS	MEANING	EXAMPLES
occipit(o)	pertaining to the occipital region of the skull	**occipito**parietal – Pertaining to the occipital and parietal bones or lobes of the skull.
ocul(o)	eye	**oculo**motor – Pertaining to movements of the eye.
		intra**ocul**ar – Within the eye.
odont(o)	tooth	orth**odont**ics – A branch of dentistry dealing with the correction of teeth.
		odontalgia – A toothache.
odyn(o)	pain	gastr**odyn**ia – Pain in the stomach.
		odynophagia – Pain when swallowing.
ole(o)	oil	**ole**aginous – To be oily or greasy.
		olearthrosis – Injection of oil into a joint.
olfact(o)	smell	**olfacto**logy – The study of the sense of smell.
		olfactory – Pertaining to the sense of smell.
olig(o)	few	**oligo**spermia – Having a small amount of sperm.
		oligodontia – Having fewer than normal teeth.
om(o)	shoulder	**om**oclavicular – Pertaining to the shoulder and clavicle.
		omohyoid – Pertaining to the shoulder and the hyoid bone.
omphal(o)	navel	**omphalo**rrhagia – Bleeding of the navel.
		omphalotomy – The cutting of the umbilical cord.
onc(o)	tumor; barb	**onco**genesis – The growth of a tumor.
		oncovirus – A virus that produces a tumor.
		oncosphere – Tapeworm larvae within embryonic envelope and armed with six hooks.
oneir(o)	dream	**oneir**ism – Waking dream state.

MEDICAL ROOTS	MEANING	EXAMPLES
onych(o)	nail	**onych**omycosis – A fungal infection of the nails.
oo(o)	egg	**oo**genesis – The development of the ova or egg.
		oocyte – An egg cell.
oophor(o)	ovary	**oophor**ectomy – Surgical removal of one or both ovaries.
		oophorocystosis – The formation of ovarian cysts.
opac(o)	not translucent; dark	**opac**ity – The state of being opaque or impervious to light.
ophthalm(o)	eye	ex**ophthalmo**s – Protrusion of the eyeball.
		ophthalmorrhea – Bleeding from the eye.
opisth(o)	backward; behind	**opistho**tonos – A spasm that causes the body to bend backwards.
		opisthognathous – Having jaws that recede backwards.
opt(o)	vision; eye	**opto**kinetic – Pertaining to the movement of the eye.
		optometer – A device for measuring vision.
or(o)	mouth	intra**or**al – Within the mouth.
		oral – Pertaining to the mouth.
orb(i)	circle	**orbi**cular – Circular; rounded.
		orbit – The bony cavity containing the eye and its vessels, nerves, and muscles.
orch(o)	testes	**orch**iopathy – A disease of the testes.
		orchiotomy – Surgical incision into a testis.
ortho(o)	straight; correct; normal	**ortho**dontics – A branch of dentistry dealing with the correction of teeth.
		orthopnea – Difficulty breathing unless one is in the upright position.

MEDICAL ROOTS	MEANING	EXAMPLES
osm(o)	smell; odor; impulse	an**osm**ia – Not having the ability to smell.
		osmophobia – The fear of odors or smells.
		osmoregulation – The maintenance of internal osmotic pressure in relation to the surrounding medium.
oste(o)	bone	**osteo**blast – A cell from which bone develops.
		osteomalacia – Softening of the bone.
ot(o)	ear	par**ot**id – The salivary gland of the ear.
		otorrhea – Discharge from the ear.
ov(o)	egg	**ov**iduct – A duct that allows the ova or egg to the leave from the ovary and pass to the uterus.
		syn**ov**ia – A fluid that resemble to white of an egg that is secreted by membranes.
ovari(o)	ovary	**ovario**centesis – The surgical puncture of an ovary.
		ovariorrhexis – The rupture of an ovary.
ox(o)	oxygen	hyp**ox**emia – A low amount of oxygen in the blood.
		oxyhemoglobin – Hemoglobin that is bound to oxygen.
pachy(o)	thick	**pachyo**nychia – Thickening of the nails.
		pachyglossia – Having a thick tongue.
pag(o)	fix	thoraco**pag**us – Conjoined twins connected in or near the sternal region.
palat(o)	palate	**palato**plegia – Paralysis of the palate.
		palatitis – Inflammation of the tongue.
palpebr(o)	eyelid	**palpebr**itis – Inflammation of the eyelid.
		palpebrate – To wink.

MEDICAL ROOTS	MEANING	EXAMPLES
pancreat(o)	pancreas	**pancreat**ectomy – Surgical excision of the pancreas.
		pancreatotropic – Having an affinity for the pancreas.
papill(o)	nipple-like; optic disk	**papillo**ma – A small, benign epithelial tumor; wart.
		papillitis – Inflammation of the optic disk.
papul(o)	papule; pimple	**papulo**sis – Formation of many papules.
		papular – Pertaining to or resembling a pimple.
pariet(o)	wall	**pariet**al – Pertaining to a wall.
		parietofrontal – Pertaining to the parietal and frontal bones.
parturi(o)	childbirth	**parturi**tion – The process of giving birth.
		parturiometer – An instrument for measuring the expulsive power of the uterus.
patell(o)	kneecap	**patell**ectomy – Surgical excision of the kneecap.
		patella – Kneecap.
path(o)	disease	**patho**logical – Related to pathology (disease).
		pathogenesis – The development of a disease.
pector(o)	chest	ex**pector**ation – To cough up mucous and phlegm from the chest.
		pectoral – Pertaining to the chest or breast.
ped(i)	child	**pedi**atrician – A physician who treats children.
ped(o)	foot	**ped**icure – Professional treatment of the feet.
		pedograph – A footprint.
pell(o)	skin	**pell**agra – Syndrome caused by niacin deficiency; causes dermatitis on sun-exposed skin, inflamed mucous membranes, diarrhea, and psychic disturbance.

MEDICAL WORD ROOTS

MEDICAL ROOTS	MEANING	EXAMPLES
pelv(i)	pelvis	**pelvi**otomy – Surgical incision of the pelvic bone.
		pelvimetry – Measurement of the pelvis.
pend(o)	hang	ap**pend**age – A suboordinate outgrowth of a structure.
		ap**pend**ix – A supplementary, accessory, or dependent part of a main structure.
pept(o)	digestion	**pepto**genic – Something that promotes digestion.
		peptic – Pertaining to digestion.
periton(e)	peritoneum	**peritone**algia – Pain in the peritoneum.
		peritonitis – Inflammation of the peritoneum.
perone(o)	fibula	**perone**al – Pertaining to the fibula.
pet(o)	move toward	centri**pet**al – Toward a center.
phac(o)	lens	**phaco**cele – Hernia of the eye lens.
		phacomalacia – Softening of the eye lens.
phag(o)	eat	**phago**cyte – A cell that ingests foreign particles.
		poly**phago**us – Eating many types of food.
phalang(o)	phalanges; fingers; toes	**phalang**ectomy – Surgical excision of a finger or toe.
		inter**phalang**eal – Between the fingers or toes.
pharmac(o)	drug	**pharmaco**logy – The study of drugs.
		pharmacognosy – The study of natural drugs.
pharyng(o)	throat; pharynx	**pharyngo**cele – A hernia of the pharynx.
		pharyngomycosis – A fungal infection of the pharynx.
phe(o)	dusky	**pheo**chrome – Stained darkly with chromium salts.

MEDICAL ROOTS	MEANING	EXAMPLES
phen(o)	show	**phen**otype – Observable characteristics of an individual.
pher(o)	support; outer edge; outside	peri**pher**y – An outward surface or structure; an outer edge.
		pheromone – Substance secreted to the outside of the body which elicits a certain behavior in other individuals of the same species.
phleb(o)	vein	**phlebo**stasis – Slow circulation of blood in the veins.
		peri**phleb**itis – Inflammation of the tissues surrounding a vein.
phlog(o)	burn	**phlog**ogenic – Causing inflammation.
phon(o)	sound	**phono**asthenia – Weakness of voice.
		phonosurgery – Surgery to enhance the voice.
phot(o)	light	**photo**phobia – The fear of light.
		photodermatitis – Inflammation of the skin caused by exposure to sunlight.
phrax(i)	wall; fence	salpingem**phrax**is – Obstruction of an auditory tube.
phren(o)	mind; diaphragm	**phreno**plegia – Paralysis of the diaphragm.
		schizo**phren**ia – A mental disorder characterized by split personalities.
phthi(a)	decay	**phthi**sis – A wasting away of the body.
phy(o)	produce; make	osteo**phy**ma – Tumor or outgrowth of a bone.
phyc(o)	seaweed	**Phyc**omycetes – Group of fungi which are common water, leaf, and bread molds.
		phycology – Study of seaweeds and other algae.
phyl(o)	group; same kind	**phyl**ogeny – Developmental history of organisms.
phys(o)	wind; inflate	**phys**ometra – Gas in the uterine cavity.
		em**phys**ema – Irregular accumulation of air in tissues or organs.

MEDICAL ROOTS	MEANING	EXAMPLES
physi(o)	nature	**physio**logy – The study of the functions of living organisms.
		physiography – The study of the earths natural features.
phyt(o)	plant	spermato**phyt**e – A group of plants that bear seeds.
		dermato**phyt**e – Fungus of the skin; a “skin plant”.
picr(o)	bitter	**picr**ic – Extremely bitter.
		picrotoxin – A bitter poison.
pil(o)	hair	e**pil**ation – To remove hair.
		pilosebaceous – Pertaining to a hair follicle and the sebaceous gland.
plant(o)	sole of the foot	**plant**ar – Pertaining to the sole of the foot.
		plantalgia – Pain in the sole of the foot.
pleth(o)	fill	**plet**hora – Excess of blood.
		plethysmograph – Instrument used for recording variations in volume of an organ, part, or limb.
pleur(o)	rib; side	**pleur**a – A membrane surrounding the lungs.
		pleurocentesis – To remove fluid from the lungs by puncturing the pleural cavity.
plex(o)	network; braid	**plex**us – A network or intertangling of nerves.
		plexiform – Resembling a plexus.
plic(o)	fold	**plic**ate – To fold into pleats.
		plication – An operation in which a structure is folded or tucked in order to shorten it.
plumb(o)	lead	**plumb**ic – Pertaining to or associated with lead.
		plumbism – Lead poisoning.

MEDICAL ROOTS	MEANING	EXAMPLES
pneum(o)	lung; breath; air	**pneumo**coniosis – A lung disease caused by the inhalation of dust.
		pneumomycosis – A fungal disease of the lungs.
pod(o)	foot	pseudo**pod** – A false foot.
		podarthritis – Inflammation of the joints of the feet.
poikil(o)	spotted; irregular; varied	**poikilo**derma – Any skin disorder characterized by patchy discolorations.
		poikilocytosis – A condition which is characterized by varied cell shapes.
pont(o)	bridge; the pons	**pont**ic – Portion of a dental bridge that takes the place of an absent tooth.
		pontine – Pertaining to the pons.
por(o)	porous; cavity formation	osteo**por**osis – A disease in which the bones are porous and fragile.
		poradenitis – Inflammation of Iliac nodes accompanied by small abscesses.
porphyr(o)	purple	**porphyr**inuria – A condition in which the urine is purple.
pos(o)	a drink	hyper**pos**ia – Punctuated, irregular increase of fluid ingestion.
		posology – Science or a system of dosage.
posit(o)	put; place	de**posit** – Sediment; inorganic matter collecting in an organ or a body.
poster(o)	back; behind	**poster**ior – Situated at the back; opposite of anterior.
		posteroanterior – Extending from the back to the front.
presby(o)	old age	**presby**opia – Poor vision due to old age.
		presbycusis – The loss of hearing that comes with old age.
press(o)	press; force	**press**or – Tending to increase blood pressure.
		pressure – Force per unit area.

MEDICAL ROOTS	MEANING	EXAMPLES
proct(o)	anus	**procto**plegia – Paralysis of the rectum.
		proctotomy – Surgical incision of the rectum.
pros(o)	front	**pros**odemic – Direct transmission of a disease from one person to another.
		prosoplasia – Abnormal differentiation of tissue; Development into a higher level of organization or function.
prosop(o)	face	**prosopo**plegia – Paralysis of the face.
		prosoposchisis – Having a facial cleft.
prostat(o)	prostate gland	**prostato**megaly – Enlargement of the prostate gland.
		prostatodynia – Pain of the prostate gland.
prote(o)	protein	**prote**inase – An enzyme that breaks down a protein.
		proteinemia – An excess of protein in the blood.
prot(o)	first	**proto**duodenum – The first part of the duodenum.
		protopathic – The part that senses pain or is affected first.
prurit(o)	itch	**prurit**us – To itch.
psamm(o)	sand	**psamm**oma – Any tumor containing psammoma bodies (round collections of calcium).
pseud(o)	fake; false	**pseudo**cyesis – A false pregnancy.
		pseudopod – A false foot.
psych(o)	mind	**psycho**logist – Someone who studies the mind.
		psychopathy – Any mental disorder.
psychr(o)	cold	**psychro**algia – A painful, cold sensation.
		psychrophilic – Being fond of or liking cold.

MEDICAL ROOTS	MEANING	EXAMPLES
ptyal(o)	saliva	**ptyal**agogue – Something that increases saliva flow.
		ptyalism – The excessive excretion of saliva.
pub(o)	adult	**pub**erty – The age when the secondary sexual characters develop allowing for the ability to sexually reproduce.
		ischio**pub**ic – Pertaining to the ischium and pubes.
pulmon(o)	lung	**pulmon**ary – Associated with the lungs.
		pulmonectomy – Surgical excision of a lung.
puls(o)	drive	pro**puls**ion – Tendency to fall forward while walking.
punct(i)	pierce	**punct**ate – Spotted as marked with points or punctures.
		punctiform – Pointed.
pur(i)	pus	sup**pur**ation – The formation of pus.
		purulent – To be associated with pus.
py(o)	pus	**py**uria – To have pus in the urine.
		spondylo**pyo**sis – The formation of pus on a vertebra.
pyg(o)	buttocks	**pyg**algia – Pain of the buttocks.
pyel(o)	pelvis; usually renal pelvis	**pyel**ectasis – Dilation of the renal pelvis.
		pyelonephritis – Inflammation of the kidney and pelvis because of a bacterial infection.
pykn(o)	thick; compact	**pykno**morphous – To stain deeply because the material being stained is deeply packed.
		pyknophasia – Having thick speech.
pyl(e)	door	**pyl**ephlebitis – Inflammation of the portal vein.
pylor(o)	pylorus	**pyloro**spasm – A spasm of the pylorus.
		pylorectomy – Surgical excision of the pylorus.

MEDICAL ROOTS	MEANING	EXAMPLES
pyr(o)	fire; heat; fever	**pyro**gen – A substance which induces a fever.
		pyromania – An obsession with fire.
radi(o)	x-ray; radius	**radi**al – Pertaining to or associated with the radius.
		radionecrosis – Tissue destruction due to x-rays.
rect(o)	rectum; straight	**recto**cele – Herniation of the rectum into the vagina.
		rectification – To make straight or correct.
ren(o)	kidney	**ren**in – An enzyme of the kidney.
		renoprival – Pertaining to a lack of kidney function.
retin(o)	retina	**retin**itis – Inflammation of the retina.
		retinoschisis – Splitting of the retina.
rhabd(o)	rod; striated	**rhabdo**myoma – A benign tumor made up of striated muscle.
		rhabdoviridae – A family of rod-shaped viruses.
rhag(o)	burst	hemor**rhag**e – The flow of blood out of the vessels; bleeding.
rhaph(o)	suture	arterior**rhaph**y – Suture of an artery.
rhe(o)	flow	diar**rhe**a – Frequent evacuation of watery feces.
rhex(i)	burst	metro**rhex**is – Rupture of the uterus.
rhin(o)	nose	**rhino**plasty – Plastic surgery of the nose.
		rhinorrhea – Discharge of fluid through the nose.
rhiz(o)	root	**rhizo**tomy – Cutting of the spinal nerve roots.
		rhizoid – To resemble a root.

MEDICAL ROOTS	MEANING	EXAMPLES
rhod(o)	rose	**rhod**amine – Group of red fluorescent dyes used to label proteins.
		rhodopsin – A photosensitive purple-red chromoprotein in the retinal rods.
rot(o)	wheel	**rot**ablation – Atherectomy technique in which a rotating burr is placed through a catheter into an artery.
		rotate – To turn around an axis.
rubr(o)	red	**rubr**ospinal – Pertaining to the red nucleus and the spinal cord.
sacr(o)	sacrum	**sacr**algia – Pain in the sacrum.
		sacrospinal – Pertaining to the sacrum and spinal column.
salping(o)	uterine tube	**salpingo**cele – Herniation of the uterine tube.
		salpingectomy – Surgical excision of the uterine tube.
sapr(o)	decay	**sapro**be – An organism that feeds on decaying matter.
		saprozoic – To live on decaying matter.
sarc(o)	flesh; connective tissue	**sarco**ma – A tumor that forms from connective tissue.
		sarcosis – The abnormal growth of flesh.
scaph(o)	small boat	**scaph**ocephaly-Condition of having an abnormally long and narrow skull.
		scaphoid – Boat-shaped; scaphoid bone.
scapul(o)	scapula	**scapulo**pexy – Surgical fixation of the scapula.
		scapulalgia – Pain of the scapular region.
scat(o)	dung	**scat**ology – Diagnostic study and analysis of feces.
schiz(o)	split; divide	**schizo**phrenia – A mental disorder characterized by split personalities.
		schizonychia – Splitting of the nails.
scirrh(o)	hard	**scirrho**us – Pertaining to hardness.

MEDICAL ROOTS	MEANING	EXAMPLES
scler(o)	hard	**sclero**derma – A hardening of the skin.
		sclerosis – The hardening of tissue.
scoli(o)	bent; crooked	**scolio**sis – A curving of the spine.
		scoliosiometry – The measurement of the curvature of the spine.
scot(o)	darkness	**scoto**phobia – An abnormal fear of the dark.
		scotopia – The ability to see in dim light.
scrot(o)	scrotum	**scroto**cele – A hernia of the scrotum.
		scrotectomy – Surgical excision of the scrotum.
seb(o)	sebaceous; fat; grease	**sebo**rrhea – An abnormal discharge from the sebaceous glands.
		sebum – The oil that is secreted through the sebaceous glands.
sect(i)	cut	bi**sect** – Cut into two parts.
		dis**sect** – Cut apart; expose structures on a cadaver for study.
semin(o)	semen; seed	**semin**uria – The presence of semen in the urine.
		in**semin**ation – To inject semen into the reproductive tract of a female.
sens(o)	perception	**sens**ible – Perceptible to the senses.
		sensory – Pertaining to sensation.
seps(o)	infection	**seps**is – An infection.
sept(o)	wall off; fence	**septo**nasal – Pertaining to the division or wall of the nose.
		septate – To be divided by a septum.
ser(o)	serum; watery substance	**sero**purulent – To be both serous and purulent.
		serosanguineous – Made up of both serum and blood.

MEDICAL ROOTS	MEANING	EXAMPLES
sial(o)	saliva	**sial**ectasia – The dilation of a salivary duct.
		sialagogue – An agent that stimulates the flow of saliva.
sider(o)	iron	**sidero**derma – A bronze discoloration of the skin caused by a problem with iron metabolism.
		siderosis – A disease of the lungs caused by inhalation of iron.
sigmoid(o)	sigmoid	**sigmoido**tomy – Surgical incision of the sigmoid colon.
		sigmoiditis – Inflammation of the sigmoid colon.
sin(o)	sinus; hollow tube	**sino**bronchitis – Inflammation of the paranasal sinus along with bronchial inflammation.
		sinoatrial – Relating to the sinoatrial node of the heart.
sinistr(o)	left	**sinistro**cular – Being dominant in the left eye.
		sinistropedal – Using the left foot over the right foot.
sit(o)	food	para**sit**e – Plant or animal that gains benefit from living in or on another organism at the organism's expense.
somat(o)	body	**somat**ic – Pertaining to the body.
		psycho**somat**ic – Pertaining to or involving both the mind and the body.
somn(o)	sleep	**somn**ambulism – Sleepwalking.
		in**somn**iac – A person who has difficulty sleeping.
son(o)	sound	**son**ication – The disruption of bacteria by exposure to sound waves that are high in frequency.
		sonogram – The image of a fetus produced by reflecting sound waves.
sopor(o)	deep sleep	**sopor**ific – To induce sleep.
		sopor – An unnaturally deep sleep.

MEDICAL WORD ROOTS

MEDICAL ROOTS	MEANING	EXAMPLES
spasm(o)	involuntary muscle contraction; draw; pull	**spasmo**lysis – To stop muscle spasms.
spectr(o)	appearance; that which is seen	**spectr**oscope – Instrument used for revealing and analyzing spectra.
sperm(at)	semen	**spermat**ogenesis – The production of sperm.
		spermicide – An agent that kills sperm.
spers(i)	scatter	a**spers**e – To sprinkle water or dust.
		di**sperse** – To scatter parts (e.g. parts of a tumor).
sphen(o)	wedge; sphenoid bone	**spheno**id – Wedge-shaped.
		sphenoiditis – Inflammation of the sphenoid sinus.
spher(o)	round; sphere-like	hemi**spher**e – Half of a globe or sphere. Also, half of the cerebrum or cerebellum.
		spherocyte – A sphere-shaped cell.
sphygm(o)	pulse	**sphygmo**manometer – An instrument that measures arterial blood pressure.
		sphygmoid – Resembling the pulse.
spin(o)	spine	**spino**cerebellar – Pertaining to the spine and the cerebellum.
		spinal – Pertaining to or associated with the spine.
spir(o)	coil; breathing	re**spir**ation – The act of breathing.
		spirochete – A microorganism that is coil-shaped.
splanchn(o)	viscera	**splanchno**logy – The study of the viscera of the body.
		splanchnicectomy – Surgical excision of one or more splanchnic nerves.
splen(o)	spleen	**spleno**megaly – Enlargement of the spleen.
		splenopexy – Surgical fixation of the spleen.

MEDICAL ROOTS	MEANING	EXAMPLES
spondyl(o)	vertebrae	**spondylo**pyosis – The formation of pus on a vertebra.
		spondylolysis – The breaking down of a vertebra.
spor(o)	seed	**spor**ocyst – Cyst or sac containing reproductive cells.
		zoo**spor**e – Motile, flagellated spore produced by algae, fungi, or protozoa.
squam(o)	scale; skin	de**squam**ation – The shedding or peeling of skin.
		squamous – Scaly.
staped(o)	stapes; stirrup-like bone of the middle ear	**staped**ectomy – Surgical removal of the stapes.
		stapedial – Pertaining to or associated with the stapes.
staphyl(o)	cluster of grapes; uvula	**staphylo**coccus – A round shaped gram-positive bacteria that is usually found in clusters like grapes.
		staphyline – Pertaining to the uvula.
stear(o)	fat	**stear**ic acid – Saturated fatty acid found in most fats or oils.
steat(o)	fat	**steato**rrhea – An excess of fat in the feces.
		steatonecrosis – The death of fatty tissue.
sten(o)	narrow	**steno**sis – The narrowing or a duct or canal.
		stenothermic – Only thriving within a certain range of temperature (e.g. bacteria).
sterc(o)	feces	**sterco**roma – A mass of fecal matter that is tumor-like.
		stercolith – A hard mass of fecal matter.
stern(o)	sternum; breastbone	**stern**algia – Pain in the sternum.
		sternoschisis – A splitting of the sternum.
steth(o)	chest	**stetho**scope – A instrument used for listening to the sounds of the chest.
		stethospasm – Spasm of the chest muscles.

MEDICAL ROOTS	MEANING	EXAMPLES
stol(o)	send	dia**stol**e – Dialation of the heart's ventricles.
		pi**stol** – The smallest firearm intended to be fired with one hand.
stomat(o)	mouth	**stomato**menia – Bleeding of the mouth during menstruation.
		stomatomalacia – A softening of the mouth.
strept(o)	twist	**strepto**coccus – A round shaped bacteria that usually occurs in pairs or strains.
strict(o)	tighten; draw tight	con**strict**ion – Narrowing or compression of a part.
stroph(o)	twist	dia**stroph**ic – Bent or curved (e.g. bones).
		strophulus – Papular hives.
struct(o)	pile up	ob**struct**ion – Blockage or clogging.
		structure – Edifice, construction, or pile.
styl(o)	stake; pillar; poke	**stylo**id – Resembling a pillar; relating to the styloid process.
		stylohyoid – Pertaining to the styloid process and hyoid bone.
sudor(i)	sweat	**sudori**parous – To produce sweat.
syring(o)	pipe; tube; fistula	**syring**itis – Inflammation of the auditory tube.
		syringectomy – Surgical excision of a fistula.
tact(o)	touch	con**tact** – The act of touching something.
		tactile – Pertaining to touch.
tal(o)	ankle bone; talus	**talo**crural – Pertaining to the talus and the leg bones.
		talofibular – Pertaining to the talus and the fibula.
tars(o)	flat surface	**tarso**ptosis – Flatfooted.
		tarsomalacia – The softening of the tarsus of an eyelid.

MEDICAL ROOTS	MEANING	EXAMPLES
taut(o)	same	**taut**omerism – Relationship between two constitutional isomers in equilibrium that can freely change from one to the other.
tax(o)	order; arrangement	a**tax**ia – Having no coordination.
		taxonomy – The grouping of organisms according to shared characteristics.
tect(i)	cover	pro**tect**in – Membrane-bound protein that prevents insertion of the membrane attack complex into the membrane.
teg(u)	cover	in**teg**ument – Covering.
tel(o)	end	**telo**phase – The final stage of mitosis.
		telomere – The end of a eukaryotic chromosome.
tempor(o)	time; the temple	**tempor**ary – Limited in time.
		temporal – Pertaining to the temple.
ten(o)	tendon	**teno**plasty – Surgical repair of a tendon.
		tenodesis – Surgical fixation of a tendon to a bone.
terat(o)	monster	**terato**ma – A tumor that is made up of different types of tissue.
		teratogen – An agent that causes abnormal prenatal development.
test(o)	testicle	**test**algia – Pain of the testicle.
		testosterone – A hormone produced by the testes.
thanat(o)	death	**thanato**phobia – An abnormal fear of death.
		thanatophoric – To be deadly or lethal.
thec(o)	sheath; case	**thec**a – A case or sheath.
		thecoma – A tumor made up of theca cells.

MEDICAL ROOTS	MEANING	EXAMPLES
thel(o)	nipple	**thel**arche – The beginning of breast development at puberty.
		thelitis – Inflammation of the nipple.
therm(o)	heat	**thermo**meter – A device that measures temperature.
		thermostabile – Not affected by heat.
the(o)	put; place	syn**the**sis – Combining simpler parts to create a whole.
thigm(o)	touch	**thigm**otaxis – Causing movement by response to contact or touch.
thorac(o)	chest	**thorac**algia – Chest pain.
		thoracostenosis – An abnormal contraction of the thorax.
thromb(o)	clot	**thrombo**cytopenia – An abnormally low number of platelets in the blood.
		thrombogenesis – Clot formation.
thym(o)	thymus gland	**thym**ectomy – Surgical excision of the thymus.
		thymocyte – A white blood cell that arises from the thymus.
thyr(o)	thyroid gland	**thyro**megaly – An enlarged thyroid gland.
		thyrotropin – Thyroid stimulating hormone.
tibi(o)	tibia	**tibio**femoral – Pertaining to the tibia and femur.
		tibiofibular – Pertaining to the tibia and fibula.
ton(o)	tone; tension	**tono**metry – The measurement of tension or pressure.
		vaso**ton**ic – Pertaining to the tension or tone of the blood vessels.
tonsill(o)	tonsils	**tonsill**itis – Inflammation of the tonsils.
		tonsillectomy – Surgical excision of a tonsil.

MEDICAL ROOTS	MEANING	EXAMPLES
top(o)	place	**top**esthesia – The ability to recognize the sensation of touch.
		topography – The description of a particular part of the body.
tors(o)	twist; rotate	**tors**ion – Twisting or rotating around an axis.
		torso – Trunk.
tort(i)	twist; rotate	**torti**collis – A twisting of the neck to one side caused by contraction of neck muscles.
		tortellini – A pasta that is twisted into a ring-like shape and stuffed with meat or cheese.
tox(o)	poison	**tox**emia – Poisoned blood caused by bacteria.
		toxicity – The state of being poisonous.
trache(o)	trachea	**tracheo**tomy – Surgical incision of the trachea through the neck.
		tracheocele – A herniation of the tracheal mucous membrane.
tract(o)	draw; drag	**tract**ion – Act of drawing or pulling.
traum(a)	wound	**traum**atism – Physical or psychic state resulting from injury.
trep(o)	turn	**trep**opnea – Difficult breathing that is relieved when the patient is lying on the side.
trich(o)	hair	**trich**iasis – A condition which causes the eyelashes to grow inward.
		trichomycosis – Any fungal disease of the hair.
trip(o)	rub	litho**trip**sy – Destruction of a calcium stone within the urinary system or gallbladder and washing away of the particles.
tub(o)	pipe	**tub**oplasty – Plastic repair of a tube (e.g. uterine or auditory).
tuber(o)	swelling; node	**tuber**cle – Nodule or small projection.
tympan(o)	eardrum	**tympano**centesis – The surgical puncture of the tympanic membrane.
		tympanoplasty – Surgical reconstruction of the tympanic membrane.

MEDICAL WORD ROOTS

MEDICAL ROOTS	MEANING	EXAMPLES
typ(o)	type	**typ**ology – Study of types; science of classifying according to type.
tyr(o)	cheese	**tyr**omatosis – Disease of caseous (resembling cheese) degeneration.
ul(o)	scar; gum	**ul**erythema – Erythematous skin disease with scarring and atrophy.
		ulotomy – Incision of scar tissue; incision of the gums.
ulcer(o)	ulcer	**ulcer**ation – The development of an ulcer.
		ulcerogenic – Something that causes or leads to ulcers.
uln(o)	ulna; elbow	**uln**ar – Pertaining to the ulna.
		ulnoradial – Pertaining the ulna and radius.
umbilic(o)	navel	**umbilic**al – Pertaining to the navel.
		umbilication – Resembling the navel.
ungu(o)	nail	sub**ungu**al – Beneath the nail.
		ungual – Pertaining to the nails.
ur(o)	urine	lith**ur**esis – Small stones in the urine.
		semin**ur**ia – The presence of semen in the urine.
ureter(o)	ureter	**ureter**ectasis – Dilation of the ureter.
		ureterolith – A calculus in the ureter.
urethr(o)	urethra	**urethro**rrhagia – The flow of blood from the urethra.
		urethrostenosis – The narrowing of the urethra.
uter(o)	uterus; womb	**utero**pexy – Surgical fixation of the uterus.
		uteropelvic – Pertaining to the uterus and the pelvis.

MEDICAL ROOTS	MEANING	EXAMPLES
uvul(o)	uvula	**uvul**itis – Inflammation of the uvula.
		uvulectomy – Surgical excision of the uvula.
vacc(a)	cow	**vacc**inia – Cowpox.
vag(o)	vagus nerve	**vago**tomy – Surgical incision of the vagus nerve.
		vagolysis – Surgical destruction of the vagus nerve.
vagin(o)	vagina	**vagino**dynia – Pain in the vagina.
		vaginitis – Inflammation of the vagina.
varic(o)	varicose vein	**varic**oblepharon – Varicose swelling of eyelid.
		varicography – X-ray visualization of varicose veins.
vas(o)	vessel	**vaso**tonic – Pertaining to the tension or tone of the blood vessels.
		vasodilation – Dilation of the blood vessels.
ven(o)	vein	**ven**ule – A small vein.
		venostasis – The stoppage of blood flow through the veins.
ventr(o)	belly	**ventro**lateral – Pertaining to the front and side.
		ventroposterior – Pertaining to the front and the back.
vertebr(o)	vertebra	in**vertebr**ate – An organism that does not have a spinal column.
		vertebrocostal – Pertaining to a vertebra and a rib.
vers(o)	turn	con**vers**ion – Change; transformation.
vert(i)	turn	in**vert** – Upside down or in the opposite position.
vesic(o)	bladder	**vesico**vaginal – Pertaining to the bladder and vagina.
		vesicle – A small sac that is filled with fluid.

MEDICAL WORD ROOTS

MEDICAL ROOTS	MEANING	EXAMPLES
vir(i)	male; masculine	**viri**le – Masculine.
		virilism – The development of male characteristics.
vir(o)	virus; poison	**vir**uria – Having viruses in the urine.
		virolactia – Secretion of viruses in milk.
viscer(o)	internal organ	**viscero**megaly – Enlargement of an internal organ.
		visceralgia – Pain of a viscera.
vit(o)	life	**vito**dynamics – Pertaining to the forces of life.
		vital – To be necessary in order to live.
vitre(o)	glassy	**vitreo**us – To have a glasslike appearance.
vuls(o)	twitch	con**vuls**ion – Involuntary contractions of voluntary muscle; seizure.
vulv(o)	vulva	**vulv**ectomy – Surgical excision of the vulva.
		vulvitis – Inflammation of the vulva.
xanth(o)	yellow	**xantho**derma – A yellowish discoloration of the skin.
		xanthochromic – To have a yellow discoloration.
xen(o)	foreign; strange	**xeno**genous – Caused by a foreign substance.
		xenophobia – An irrational fear of strangers.
xer(o)	dry	**xero**derma – To have dry skin.
		xeroma – A dryness of the conjunctiva of the eye.
xiph(o)	sword; xiphoid process	**xipho**iditis – Inflammation of the xiphoid process.
		xiphocostal – Pertaining to the xiphoid process and the ribs.

MEDICAL ROOTS	MEANING	EXAMPLES
zyg(o)	union; yoke	**zyg**ote – The union of two gametes or a fertilized egg.
		zygosis – Conjugation.
zym(o)	ferment; catalyst; enzyme	en**zym**e – Any protein that functions as a biological catalyst.
		zymosis – Fermentation.

Medical Suffixes

"The artist is nothing without the gift, but the gift is nothing without work."

– Emile Zola

SUFFIXES

MEDICAL SUFFIXES	MEANING	EXAMPLES
-ac	pertaining or referring to	cardi**ac** – Relating to the heart.
		mani**ac** – An individual who experiences mania.
-ad	toward; add; group; connection	caud**ad** – Toward the cauda (tail). In the human, this corresponds with the coccyx bone at the distal inferior end of the vertebral column.
		Trichomon**ad** – Parasite of genus *Trichomonas.*
-agogue	an entity or event that stimulates, causes, or induces	syn**agogue** – A Jewish place of worship.
		antisial**agogue** – An agent that causes a decreased secretion of saliva.
-agra	seizure; pain	pod**agra** – Pain in the foot caused by gout.
-al	pertaining to; act; process	femor**al** – Associated with the femur bone. (e.g. femoral nerve)
		pathologic**al** – Related to pathology (disease).
		refus**al** – The act of denial.
-algia	pain	my**algia** – Pain of one or more muscles.
		arthr**algia** – Pain of one or more joints.
-ar	relating or pertaining to	cardiovascul**ar** – Related to the heart and vasculature.
		follicul**ar** – Related to one or more follicles.
-arch(e)	first; origin	patri**arch** – A man considered to be a father or founder.
		men**arche** – The onset of menstruation.
-ary	pertaining to or associated with	pulmon**ary** – Associated with the lungs.
		integument**ary** – Associated with the integument (the skin).
-ase	a suffix denoting an enzyme	protein**ase** – An enzyme that breaks down a protein.
		lip**ase** – An enzyme that breaks down a fat.
-asthenia	weakness; loss of strength	my**asthenia** – Muscular weakness (e.g. myasthenia gravis).

MEDICAL SUFFIXES	MEANING	EXAMPLES
-blast	pertaining to a cell in the early stages of growth	osteo**blast** – A cell from which bone develops.
		melano**blast** – A cell that develops into a melanocyte.
-capnia	carbon dioxide	hyper**capnia** – Excessive amounts of carbon dioxide in the lungs.
-cele	hernia; tumor; hollow	myo**cele** – Protrusion of muscle.
		aero**cele** – An air-filled pouch, particularly one attached to the trachea or larynx.
-centesis	puncture	amnio**centesis** – The surgical procedure of inserting a needle through the abdominal wall and uterus to obtain amniotic fluid for tests.
		entero**centesis** – Surgical puncture of the intestine to withdraw gas or fluid.
-cept	receive	inter**cept** – Prevent someone or something from continuing to its destination.
		re**cept**or – A region of tissue, or a molecule on a cell surface, that responds specifically to a certain neurotransmitter, hormone, antigen, or other substance.
-cid(e)	kill	fungi**cide** – A chemical that kills fungi.
		bacteri**cid**al – Something that kills bacteria.
-clast	break	osteo**clast** – A cell that breaks down bone.
		icono**clast** – A person who seeks to break or destroy popular ideas.
-cleisis	enclose	colpo**cleisis** – Surgical closure of the vaginal cavity.
-coccus	berry	staphylo**coccus** – A round shaped gram-positive bacteria that is usually found in clusters like grapes.
		strepto**coccus** – A round shaped bacteria that usually occurs in pairs or strains.
-crasia	mixture	dys**crasia** – An abnormal mixture of the blood.
-crescence	growth	ex**crescence** – Anything growing out unnaturally from anything else such as a wart or tumor.
		con**crescence** – Growing together of parts that were orignially separate.

MEDICAL SUFFIXES	MEANING	EXAMPLES
-crine	secrete	endo**crine** – Secretion of hormones internally into the blood.
		exo**crine** – Secretion of hormones externally into a duct.
-cusis	hearing	ana**cusis** – Completely deaf.
		presby**cusis** – The loss of hearing the comes with old age.
-cyesis	pregnancy	pseudo**cyesis** – A false pregnancy.
-cyte	cell	leuko**cyte** – White blood cell.
		erythro**cyte** – Red blood cell.
-desis	binding together	arthro**desis** – A surgical procedure which immobilizes a joint.
		syn**desis** – To bind together.
-ducent	lead; tube; duct	ab**ducent** – Serving to draw toward the medial plane or toward the axial line of a limb.
		ad**ducent** – Serving to draw away from the medial plane or from the axial line of a limb.
-ectasia	dilation; expansion	tangi**ectasia** – Dark red blotches on the skin that are caused by abnormal dilation of groups of capillaries.
		col**ectasia** – Dilation of the colon.
-ectomy	to take out	append**ectomy** – Surgical excision of the vermiform appendix.
		hyster**ectomy** – Surgical excision of the uterus.
-emesis	vomit	hyper**emesis** – Excessive vomiting.
		hemat**emesis** – Vomiting blood.
-emia	blood	an**emia** – Lack of red blood cells.
		septic**emia** – Pathogenic bacteria in the bloodstream; blood poisoning.
-esis	act; process	gen**esis** – The act or process of originating or giving birth.
		cytokin**esis** – Final stage of cell division when the cytoplasm splits.

MEDICAL SUFFIXES	MEANING	EXAMPLES
-facient	make	cale**facient** – That which causes warmth.
		aborti**facient** – That which causes a miscarriage.
-fect	make	af**fect** – A show of emotion; to produce an effect.
		in**fect**ious – Caused by or capable of being transmitted by an infection.
-ferent	bear; carry	ef**ferent** – Carrying away from an organ or part.
		de**ferent** – Serving to carry.
-ferous	to bear	lacti**ferous** – To bear or contain milk.
		somni**ferous** – To induce sleep.
-form	shape	uni**form** – Having the same shape.
-genesis	origin; generation	carcino**genesis** – The growth of cancer.
		oo**genesis** – The development of the ova.
-globin	protein	hemo**globin** – A protein found in red blood cells.
		myo**globin** – A protein found in the muscle.
-grade	movement; walk; go	retro**grade** – To go backwards.
		up**grade** – To go upwards.
-gram	drawing; record; letter	cardio**gram** – A drawing of the cardiac cycle used to diagnose heart disorders.
		tele**gram** – A message sent by telegraph.
-graph	record; write	calli**graph**er – Fancy writing.
		baro**graph** – An instrument that records the atmospheric pressure.
-ia	state; condition; quality of	eupeps**ia** – Good or normal digestion.
		anem**ia** – Lack of red blood cells.

MEDICAL SUFFIXES	MEANING	EXAMPLES
-iasis	condition; state of; disease	cholelith**iasis** – Formation of stones in the biliary system.
		mydr**iasis** – Excessive dilation of the pupil.
-ic	associated with; pertaining to	geriatr**ic**s – Medicine that deals with the elderly.
-id	form; resemblance	lipo**id** – To resemble fat.
		plast**id** – Any of a class of small organelles in the cytoplasm of plant cells, containing pigment or food.
-ism	a suffix which makes the word a noun	alcohol**ism** – Disorder marked by alcohol abuse.
		isomer**ism** – Two compounds with the same number of atoms of each element, but in different arrangement.
-ist	a person who practices	scient**ist** – Someone who practices science.
		psycholog**ist** – Someone who practices psychology.
-itis	inflammation	cyst**itis** – Inflammation of the bladder.
		bronch**itis** – Inflammation of one or more bronchi.
-ize	a suffix which makes the word a verb	cauter**ize** – To destroy tissue by application with heat, cold, or a caustic agent.
		oxid**ize** – Cause to bond with oxygen or remove hydrogen.
-ject	throw	inter**ject** – To speak abruptly; an interruption.
-lemma	husk; outer shell	sarco**lemma** – The membrane of a striated muscle cell.
-lepsy	seizure; attack; uncontrolled	narco**lepsy** – A disorder that causes uncontrolled episodes of deep sleep.
		epi**lepsy** – A disorder of the nervous system that causes brain malfunction and often results in seizures.
-logy	study of	immuno**logy** – The study of the immune system.
		nephro**logy** – The study of the kidneys.

MEDICAL SUFFIXES	MEANING	EXAMPLES
-lysis	breakdown; split; dissolution	lipo**lysis** – The breakdown of fat.
		hydro**lysis** – The splitting of water molecules.
-lytic	breakdown; destruction	ana**lytic**al – Pertaining to the breakdown of thoughts.
		hemo**lytic** – The breakdown of red blood cells.
-malacia	softening	osteo**malacia** – Softening of the bone.
		encephalo**malacia** – Softening of the brain.
-megaly	enlarged	acro**megaly** – Enlargement of the extremities of the body (fingers, nose, jaw) by excessive growth hormone.
		cephalo**megaly** – Enlargement of the head.
-mer	part	poly**mer** – A compound formed by combination of simpler molecules.
-meter	measurement	thermo**meter** – A device that measures temperature.
		baro**meter** – An instrument for measuring weight or pressure of the atmosphere.
-mimetic	mimic; copy	sympatho**mimetic** – To mimic the effects caused by stimulation of the sympathetic nervous system.
		radio**mimetic** – Having similar effect to radiation.
-mittent	send	inter**mittent** – Alternating periods of activity and inactivity.
		re**mittent** – As of a fever with fluctuating body temperatures.
-nychia	nail	pachyo**nychia** – Thickening of the nails.
		ano**nychia** – Not having fingernails.
-ode	road, path, resemblance	cath**ode** – The electric node to which positive charge is attracted.
		nemat**ode** – Roundworm.

MEDICAL SUFFIXES	MEANING	EXAMPLES
-oid	resembling; like; equivalent	lip**oid** – To resemble fat.
		choan**oid** – Funnel-shaped.
-ol	oil	choleste**rol** – Sterol precursor of bile acids and steroid hormones and a component of cell membranes.
-ole	small; little	arteri**ole** – A small artery.
		bronchi**ole** – A small extension of a bronchus.
-oma	tumor	hemangi**oma** – A tumor made up of blood vessels.
		carcin**oma** – A cancerous tumor.
-on	goes; moves	electr**on** – Negatively charged particle.
		positr**on** – Positively charged particle.
-opia	vision	dipl**opia** – Having double vision.
-opsia	vision	cyan**opsia** – A problem with the eye that causes things to appear blue.
-opsy	to view	aut**opsy** – To inspect a body after death to determine the cause.
		bi**opsy** – To examine a piece of tissue from the body for diagnosis.
-orrhagia	profuse bleeding	omphal**orrhagia** – Bleeding of the navel.
		men**orrhagia** – Profuse bleeding from the uterus.
-orrhea	flow; discharge	metr**orrhea** – An abnormal discharge from the uterus.
		galact**orrhea** – Excessive flow of milk.
-osis	process; disorder; disease	dyshidr**osis** – A disorder of the sweat glands.
		dermat**osis** – A disease of the skin.
-ostomy	mouth; artificial or surgical opening	col**ostomy** – A surgical operation to create an artificial anus.
		gastrojejun**ostomy** – Surgery to make a new passage between the stomach and jejunum.

MEDICAL SUFFIXES	MEANING	EXAMPLES
-otomy	cut; incision	crani**otomy** – Surgery in which the skull is opened.
		hyster**otomy** – Surgical incision of the uterus through either the abdomen or vagina.
-ous	pertaining or referring to; full of; abounding	aque**ous** – Full of water.
		frivol**ous** – Very carefree; not serious.
-para	birth	nulli**para** – A woman who has never given birth to a child.
		primi**para** – A woman who is pregnant for the first time.
-paresis	partial paralysis	hemi**paresis** – Partial paralysis of one half of the body.
		gastro**paresis** – A partial paralysis of the stomach.
-partum	birth	post-**partum** – Occurring after birth.
-pathy	disease	orchio**pathy** – A disease of the testes.
		hystero**pathy** – A disease of the uterus.
-penia	decrease; deficiency	erythro**penia** – A low number of red blood cells.
		leuko**penia** – A low number of white blood cells.
-pepsia	digestion	eu**pepsia** – Good or normal digestion.
		dys**pepsia** – Difficult digestion.
-pexy	to fasten; fixation	gastro**pexy** – Fixation of the stomach.
		hepato**pexy** – Fixation of the liver to the abdominal wall.
-phagia	eating	oligo**phagia** – Eating only a few types of food.
		hyper**phagia** – Constantly hungry.
-phasia	speech	a**phasia** – The inability to speak.
		dys**phasia** – Difficulty speaking.

MEDICAL SUFFIXES	MEANING	EXAMPLES
-pheresis	remove	plasma**pheresis** – To remove plasma from the blood.
-phil	like; affinity for	achromato**phil** – Not having an affinity for stain; not easily stainable.
		acido**phil** – A cell or structure easily stainable with acid dyes.
-philia	like; affinity for	hydro**philia** – Having an affinity for water.
		necro**philia** – Having a sexual attraction to dead bodies.
-phobia	fear; dread	necro**phobia** – Fear of death or dead bodies.
		gyne**phobia** – Fear of women.
-phoresis	support; bear; carry	electro**phoresis** – Transmission of electrical current.
		dia**phoresis** – Perspiration; secretion of sweat.
-phoria	mood; feeling	eu**phoria** – To be happy; content.
		dys**phoria** – Not satisfied; impatient.
-phragm	wall; fence; stop up	dia**phragm** – A wall that separates two cavities in the body.
-phylaxis	protection	chemopro**phylaxis** – Protection against disease by means of chemicals agents.
-phyll	leaf	chloro**phyll** – Group of porphyrin derivatives that contain green magnesium; necessary for photosynthesis.
-physis	growth	apo**physis** – An outgrowth. Often used to describe bony outgrowths that do not separate from the bone (e.g. tubercle process).
		sym**physis** – To grow together.
-plasia	formation; growth	hyper**plasia** – Excessive growth.
		achondro**plasia** – Improper growth of cartilage.
-plasm	formation; growth substance	neo**plasm** – A new and abnormal growth.
		nucleo**plasm** – The protoplasm found in the nucleus of a cell.

MEDICAL SUFFIXES	MEANING	EXAMPLES
-plasty	mold; shape; surgical repair	mento**plasty** – Plastic surgery on the chin.
		chiro**plasty** – Plastic surgery on the hand.
-plegia	paralysis	logo**plegia** – Paralysis of speech organs.
		irido**plegia** – Paralysis of the sphincter of the iris.
-pnea	breath; respiration	ortho**pnea** – Difficulty breathing unless one is in the upright position.
		dys**pnea** – Difficulty breathing.
-poiesis	produce; make	leuko**poiesis** – The formation of white blood cells.
		hemato**poiesis** – The formation of blood.
-poietic	formation of	sarco**poietic** – The formation of muscle.
		myelo**poietic** – The formation of bone marrow.
-porosis	porous; cavity formation	osteo**porosis** – A disease in which the bones are porous and fragile.
-ptosis	fall; droop	nephro**ptosis** – To have a floating kidney.
		apo**ptosis** – Programmed cell death.
-ptysis	spitting	hemo**ptysis** – To spit up blood.
-salpinx	fallopian tube	pyo**salpinx** – The accumulation of pus in a fallopian tube.
-sclerosis	hardening	arterio**sclerosis** – Hardening of the arteries.
		arteriolo**sclerosis** – Hardening of arterioles.
-scope	to examine	endo**scope** – An instrument for viewing an inner part of the body.
		stetho**scope** – A instrument used for listening to the sounds of the chest.
-sis	action	diagno**sis** – Act of diagnosing.
-stalsis	contraction	per**istalsis** – Contraction of the intestines to help in food digestion.

MEDICAL SUFFIXES	MEANING	EXAMPLES
-stasis	to stop; stagnation	hemo**stasis** – The stoppage of blood flow.
		chole**stasis** – The stoppage of bile flow.
-sthenia	strength	mya**sthenia** – A lack of muscular strength.
		eu**sthenia** – Having normal strength.
-stringent	tighten; draw tight	a**stringent** – Causing contraction.
-therapy	treatment	tele**therapy** – Treatment in which the agent does not contact the body.
		chemo**therapy** – Treatment of disease through the use of chemicals.
-thorax	chest	hemo**thorax** – The presence of blood in the chest.
		pneumo**thorax** – The presence of air or gas in the chest.
-tocia	birth	dys**tocia** – To have a difficult childbirth.
		brady**tocia** – To have a slow childbirth.
-tome	a cutting instrument	derma**tome** – An instrument that is used to cut thin layers of skin.
		osteo**tome** – An instrument that is used to cut bone.
-trophy	nurture; growth; nutrition	hyper**trophy** – An excessive growth or enlargement.
		a**trophy** – To decrease in size or waste away.
-tropia	turn	eso**tropia** – The turning inward of one eye.
		exo**tropia** – The turning outward of one eye.
-ule	small; little	ven**ule** – A small vein.
		cell**ule** – A small cell.

All Medical Random Combining Forms

"We make a living by what we get.
We make a life by what we give."

– Sir Winston Churchill

RANDOM

MEDICAL ROOTS / PREFIXES / SUFFIXES	MEANING	EXAMPLES
presby(o)	old age	**presbyo**pia – Poor vision due to old age.
		presbycusis – The loss of hearing that comes with old age.
vacc(a)	cow	**vacc**inia – Cowpox.
blenn-	mucus	**blenn**orrhea – The discharge or mucus.
-meter	measurement	thermo**meter** – A device that measures temperature.
		baro**meter** – An instrument for measuring weight or pressure of the atmosphere.
aort(o)	aorta	**aort**algia – Pain in or near the aorta.
		aortopathy – A disease of the aorta.
-desis	binding together	arthro**desis** – A surgical procedure which immobilizes a joint.
		syn**desis** – To bind together.
caud(o)	tail	**caud**ad – Toward the cauda (tail). In the human, this corresponds with the coccyx bone at the distal inferior end of the vertebral column.
		caudate – Having a tail.
-al	pertaining to; act; process	femor**al** – Associated with the femur bone. (e.g. femoral nerve)
		pathologic**al** – Related to pathology (disease).
		refus**al** – The act of denial.
glauc(o)	glaucoma	**glauco**matous – Pertaining to or associated with glaucoma.
-blast	pertaining to a cell in the early stages of growth	osteo**blast** – A cell from which bone develops.
		melano**blast** – A cell that develops into a melanocyte.

MEDICAL ROOTS / PREFIXES / SUFFIXES	MEANING	EXAMPLES
olfact(o)	smell	**olfacto**logy – The study of the sense of smell.
		olfactory – Pertaining to the sense of smell.
por(o)	porous; cavity formation	osteo**por**osis – A disease in which the bones are porous and fragile.
		poradenitis – Inflammation of Iliac nodes accompanied by small abscesses.
axon(o)	the axis	**axon** – The appendage of a neuron through which nerve signals are sent.
		axonometer – A device that estimates the axis of a lens.
perone(o)	fibula	**perone**al – Pertaining to the fibula.
actin(o)	ray	**actino**dermatitis – Radiodermatitis.
		actinotherapy – Treatment with ultraviolet rays.
gen(o)	begin; originate; produce	carcino**gen**ic – A cancer producing agent.
		generation – Reproduction.
vitre(o)	glassy	**vitreo**us – To have a glasslike appearance.
duct(o)	lead; tube; duct	ab**duct** – Lead away from the medial plane.
		ovi**duct** – A duct that allows the ova or egg to the leave from the ovary and pass to the uterus.
-stalsis	contraction	peri**stalsis** – Contraction of the intestines to help in food digestion.
atri(o)	chamber that provides entrance into another location (often atrium)	right **atri**um – Provides entrance into the right ventricle of the heart.
		atriomegaly – Irregular enlargement of an atrium.
primi-	first	**primi**para – A woman who is pregnant for the first time.
		primitive – Pertaining to the first or early times.

MEDICAL ROOTS / PREFIXES / SUFFIXES	MEANING	EXAMPLES
morph(o)	shape; form	**morpho**logy – The study of shape and form.
		zoo**morph**ic – Having the form of an animal.
celi(o)	abdomen	**celio**ma – A tumor of the abdomen.
		celiac – Associated with the abdomen.
pell(o)	skin	**pell**agra – Syndrome caused by niacin deficiency; causes dermatitis on sun-exposed skin, inflamed mucous membranes, diarrhea, and psychic disturbance.
aer(o)	pertaining or referring to air	**aero**be – A microorganism that lives in oxygen exposed environments.
		aeropathy – A disease process related to a change in atmospheric pressure.
nas(o)	nose	para**nas**al – Adjacent to the nose.
		nasopharynx – The part of the pharynx that is continuous with the nasal passages.
quadri-	four	**quadri**ceps – A muscle with four heads.
		quadrigeminal – To have four parts.
macro-	large; long	**macro**melia – Having one or more limbs that are enlarged.
		macropsia – A visual disorder that causes objects to appear larger than they actually are.
rachi-	spine	**rachi**odynia – Pain of the spine.
		rachicentesis – A lumbar puncture.
immun(o)	resistance; protection	**immuni**zation – To make immune or resistant to, particularly by innoculation.
		immunosuppressant – To prevent an immune response.

MEDICAL ROOTS / PREFIXES / SUFFIXES	MEANING	EXAMPLES
abdomin(o)	referring or pertaining to the abdomen	**abdomino**hysterectomy – A surgical procedure in which an abdominal approach is used to remove the uterus.
		abdominopelvic cavity – The cavity that includes the abdominal and pelvic cavities and is surrounded by the same serrous membrane, the peritoneum.
-therapy	treatment	tele**therapy** – Treatment in which the agent does not contact the body.
		chemo**therapy** – Treatment of disease through the use of chemicals.
plant(o)	sole of the foot	**plant**ar – Pertaining to the sole of the foot.
		plantalgia – Pain in the sole of the foot.
lacrim(o)	tears; tear duct	**lacrim**ator – Something that induces the flow of tears.
		lacrimotomy – Surgical incision of the lacrimal duct or sac.
pariet(o)	wall	**pariet**al – Pertaining to a wall.
		parietofrontal – Pertaining to the parietal and frontal bones.
vag(o)	vagus nerve	**vago**tomy – Surgical incision of the vagus nerve.
		vagolysis – Surgical destruction of the vagus nerve.
campt(o)	bent	**campto**dactyly – Having a permanently bent finger.
		camptomelia – A bending of the limbs that is permanent.
hyps(o)	height	**hyps**okinesis – A swaying or falling when in erect posture.
-otomy	cut; incision	crani**otomy** – Surgery in which the skull is opened.
		hyster**otomy** – Surgical incision of the uterus through either the abdomen or vagina.

MEDICAL ROOTS / PREFIXES / SUFFIXES	MEANING	EXAMPLES
olig(o)	few	**oligo**spermia – Having a small amount of sperm.
		oligodontia – Having fewer than normal teeth.
aden(o)	pertaining or referring to a gland	**adeno**carcinoma – Carcinoma that originated from cells of glands.
		adenopathy – An increase in the size of glands often referring to lymph nodes.
sit(o)	food	para**sit**e – Plant or animal that gains benefit from living in or on another organism at the organism's expense.
trich(o)	hair	**trich**iasis – A condition which causes the eyelashes to grow inward.
		trichomycosis – Any fungal disease of the hair.
lact(o)	milk	**lacto**bacillus – A bacteria found in milk.
		lactogen – Something that enhances milk production.
therm(o)	heat	**thermo**meter – A device that measures temperature.
		thermostabile – Not affected by heat.
cerebr(o)	brain	**cerebr**um – The main portion of the brain.
		cerebrospinal – Pertaining to the brain and spinal cord.
mer(o)	thigh	**mer**algia – Pain of the thigh.
dacry(o)	tear; lacrimal gland of the eye	**dacryo**ps – An excess of tears.
		dacryoadenalgia – Pain of the lacrimal gland.
capit(a)	head	de**capit**ate – To cut off the head.
		capitate – Head-shaped.
hemangi(o)	blood vessel	**hemangio**ma – A tumor made up of blood vessels.
		hemangioblast – A developing cell that gives rise to blood vessels.

MEDICAL ROOTS / PREFIXES / SUFFIXES	MEANING	EXAMPLES
-poiesis	produce; make	leuko**poiesis** – The formation of white blood cells.
		hemato**poiesis** – The formation of blood.
radi(o)	x-ray; radius	**radi**al – Pertaining to or associated with the radius.
		radionecrosis – Tissue destruction due to x-rays.
mel(o)	limb; cheek	sym**mel**ia – A developmental anomaly characterized by a fusion of the lower limbs.
		meloplasty – Plastic sugery of the cheek.
-lytic	breakdown; destruction	ana**lytic**al – Pertaining to the breakdown of thoughts.
		hemo**lytic** – The breakdown of red blood cells.
ortho(o)	straight; correct; normal	**ortho**dontics – A branch of dentistry dealing with the correction of teeth.
		orthopnea – Difficulty breathing unless one is in the upright position.
pylor(o)	pylorus	**pyloro**spasm – A spasm of the pylorus.
		pylorectomy – Surgical excision of the pylorus.
an-	without, not	**an**oxia – Without oxygen.
		anesthesia – The loss of sensation.
vertebr(o)	vertebra	in**vertebr**ate – An organism that does not have a spinal column.
		vertebrocostal – Pertaining to a vertebra and a rib.
coel-	hollow	**coel**om – Body cavity.
		coelozoic – Living in the intestinal canal of the body.
-oma	tumor	hemangi**oma** – A tumor made up of blood vessels.
		carcin**oma** – A cancerous tumor.

MEDICAL ROOTS / PREFIXES / SUFFIXES	MEANING	EXAMPLES
ante-	forward	**ante**rior – A direction or location toward the front (opposite of posterior).
		antenna – One of the two forward appendages on the head of arthropods.
-tome	a cutting instrument	derma**tome** – An instrument that is used to cut thin layers of skin.
		osteo**tome** – An instrument that is used to cut bone.
ptyal(o)	saliva	**ptyal**agogue – Something that increases saliva flow.
		ptyalism – The excessive excretion of saliva.
-lysis	breakdown; split; dissolution	lipo**lysis** – The breakdown of fat.
		hydro**lysis** – The splitting of water molecules.
tri-	three	**tri**cep – A muscle with three heads.
		tricuspid – Having three points or cusps.
pykn(o)	thick; compact	**pykno**morphous – To stain deeply because the material being stained is deeply packed.
		pyknophasia – Having thick speech.
sens(o)	perception	**sens**ible – Perceptible to the senses.
		sensory – Pertaining to sensation.
acetabul(o)	pertaining or relating to the hip socket, by describing it as a “vinegar cup”	**acetabul**um – The cup-shaped socket of the hip joint.
		acetabuloplasty – Surgical repair of the acetabulum.
vermi-	worm	**vermi**cular – Resembling a worm.
		vermiculation – To move like a worm.

MEDICAL ROOTS / PREFIXES / SUFFIXES	MEANING	EXAMPLES
pod(o)	foot	pseudo**pod** – A false foot.
		podarthritis – Inflammation of the joints of the feet.
-trophy	nurture; growth; nutrition	hyper**trophy** – An excessive growth or enlargement.
		a**trophy** – To decrease in size or waste away.
cry(o)	cold	**cryo**anesthesia – Anesthesia caused by chilling to a near freezing temperature.
		cryogenic – Very low temperatures.
-emesis	vomit	hyper**emesis** – Excessive vomiting.
		hemat**emesis** – Vomiting blood.
nos(o)	disease	**nos**ocomial – Pertaining to or coming from a hospital (often referring to diseases transmitted in hospitals).
		nosology – Scientific classification of diseases.
allo-	other; different	**allo**rhythmia – Having an irregular heartbeat.
		allosome – A foreign part of the cytoplasm in a cell that entered from the outside.
ventr(o)	belly	**ventro**lateral – Pertaining to the front and side.
		ventroposterior – Pertaining to the front and the back.
hepat(o)	liver	**hepat**itis – Inflammation of the liver.
		hepatomegaly – Enlargement of the liver.
struct(o)	pile up	ob**struct**ion – Blockage or clogging.
		structure – Edifice, construction, or pile.
zym(o)	ferment; catalyst; enzyme	en**zym**e – Any protein that functions as a biological catalyst.
		zymosis – Fermentation.

MEDICAL ROOTS / PREFIXES / SUFFIXES	MEANING	EXAMPLES
nat(i)	birth	neo**nat**al – Pertaining to a newborn child.
		natalitial – Associated with or pertaining to a birth or birthday.
chrys(o)	gold	**chryso**derma – A permanent change in pigmentation of the skin due to gold deposits.
		chrysotherapy – Treatment with gold salts.
lith(o)	stone	nephro**litho**tripsy – Removal of kidney stones.
		lithuresis – Small stones in the urine.
home(o)	like; resembling; constant	**homeo**stasis – Staying in a constant state; equilibrium.
		homeothermy – The maintaining of constant body temperature.
co-	with; together	**co**hesion – The intermolecular force which causes particles of a material to unite.
		cohort – A group of individuals sharing a common characteristic.
papul(o)	papule; pimple	**papulo**sis – Formation of many papules.
		papular – Pertaining to or resembling a pimple.
adip(o)	pertaining or referring to fat	**adipo**cyte – A fat cell.
		adipsuria – Fat in the urine.
-ist	a person who practices	scient**ist** – Someone who practices science.
		psycholog**ist** – Someone who practices psychology.
dipl(o)	double	**diplo**pia – Seeing two of a single object.
		diploid – Having two sets of chromosomes.
medi-	middle	**medi**an – Situated in the midline of a body or structure.

MEDICAL ROOTS / PREFIXES / SUFFIXES	MEANING	EXAMPLES
tars(o)	flat surface	**tarso**ptosis – Flatfooted.
		tarsomalacia – The softening of the tarsus of an eyelid.
ox(o)	oxygen	hyp**ox**emia – A low amount of oxygen in the blood.
		oxyhemoglobin – Hemoglobin that is bound to oxygen.
ab-	away from	**ab**duct – A motion in which a structure is moved away from the midline of the body.
		abrasion – Tissue is scraped away from the skin or mucous membrane.
thanat(o)	death	**thanato**phobia – An abnormal fear of death.
		thanatophoric – To be deadly or lethal.
cycl(o)	circle; ciliary body of the eye	**cyclo**ne – A rotating windstorm; tornado.
		cyclotomy – Surgical incision of the ciliary muscle.
thel(o)	nipple	**thel**arche – The beginning of breast development at puberty.
		thelitis – Inflammation of the nipple.
chrom(o)	color	a**chrom**asia – Hypopigmentation; lack of staining power in a cell or tissue.
		chromoblast – Embryonic cell that develops into a pigment cell.
fet(o)	fetus	**feto**metry – Measurement of the fetus.
		fetology – A branch of medicine dealing with the fetus.
amni(o)	pertaining to the membrane surrounding the fetus (i.e. amnion)	**amnio**tic fluid – Fluid surrounding the fetus.
		amniocentesis – The surgical procedure of inserting a needle through the abdominal wall and uterus to obtain amniotic fluid for tests.

MEDICAL ROOTS / PREFIXES / SUFFIXES	MEANING	EXAMPLES
pyel(o)	pelvis; usually renal pelvis	**pyel**ectasis – Dilation of the renal pelvis.
		pyelonephritis – Inflammation of the kidney and pelvis because of a bacterial infection.
coni(o)	dust	**conio**sis – A disease caused by dust.
		pneumo**conio**sis – A lung disease caused by the inhalation of dust.
gamet(o)	marriage; reproduction	**gamet**e – One of two haploid reproductive cells, male or female; malarial parasite in its sexual form.
		gametogenesis – Development of the male and female sex cells.
semi-	half	**semi**circle – Half of a circle.
		semicoma – A coma in which the patient can be aroused.
acr(o)	extremity; top	**acro**megaly – Enlargement of the extremities of the body (fingers, nose, jaw) by excessive growth hormone.
		acromion – The part of the scapula bone that forms the highest part of the shoulder.
em-	in; on	**em**bedding – To fix into something.
		emphysema – A condition caused by build up of air in tissues or organs.
staped(o)	stapes; stirrup-like bone of the middle ear	**staped**ectomy – Surgical removal of the stapes.
		stapedial – Pertaining to or associated with the stapes.
tempor(o)	time; the temple	**tempor**ary – Limited in time.
		temporal – Pertaining to the temple.

MEDICAL ROOTS / PREFIXES / SUFFIXES	MEANING	EXAMPLES
omni-	every; all	**omni**potent – Having all power.
		omnivore – A person or animal that eats all kinds of foods.
parturi(o)	childbirth	**parturi**tion – The process of giving birth.
		parturiometer – An instrument for measuring the expulsive power of the uterus.
atel(o)	incomplete or imperfect	**atel**ectasis – Incomplete expansion of the lungs.
		atelocardiac – Abnormal development of the heart.
calor(o)	heat	**calor**imeter – An instrument for measuring heat.
		calorie – A unit of heat.
junct(o)	join	con**junct**iva – Membrane covering the eyeball.
ovari(o)	ovary	**ovario**centesis – The surgical puncture of an ovary.
		ovariorrhexis – The rupture of an ovary.
pneum(o)	lung; breath; air	**pneumo**coniosis – A lung disease caused by the inhalation of dust.
		pneumomycosis – A fungal disease of the lungs.
gnath(o)	jaw	**gnatho**schisis – Cleft jaw.
		a**gnath**a – A class of jawless chordates.
pont(o)	bridge; the pons	**pont**ic – Portion of a dental bridge that takes the place of an absent tooth.
		pontine – Pertaining to the pons.
-agogue	an entity or event that stimulates, causes, or induces	syn**agogue** – A Jewish place of worship.
		antisial**agogue** – An agent that causes a decreased secretion of saliva.

MEDICAL ROOTS / PREFIXES / SUFFIXES	MEANING	EXAMPLES
kerat(o)	horn-like; cornea	**kerat**in – A protein that makes up horny tissues of the body.
		keratocentesis – Puncture of the cornea.
chor(o)	membrane	**chor**ion – The outer membrane surrounding the embryo in reptiles, birds, and mammals.
		choroid – A membrane that coats the eye that is found between the sclera and the retina.
py(o)	pus	**py**uria – To have pus in the urine.
		spondylo**pyo**sis – The formation of pus on a vertebra.
lal(o)	talk	glosso**lal**ia – Nosense talk that mirrors coherent speech.
		lallation – Infantile speech.
erythr(o)	red	**erythro**cyte – Red blood cell.
ili(o)	pertaining or referring to the ilium or hip bone	**ili**ac – Referring to the hip bone.
		iliocostal – Connecting or referring to the hip bone and ribs.
-asthenia	weakness; loss of strength	my**asthenia** – Muscular weakness (e.g. myasthenia gravis).
hyster(o)	uterus; womb	**hyster**ectomy – Surgical excision of the uterus.
		hysteropathy – A disease of the uterus.
-cid(e)	kill	fungi**cide** – A chemical that kills fungi.
		bacteri**cid**al – Something that kills bacteria.
-ptosis	fall; droop	nephro**ptosis** – To have a floating kidney.
		apo**ptosis** – Programmed cell death.
-mer	part	poly**mer** – A compound formed by combination of simpler molecules.

MEDICAL ROOTS / PREFIXES / SUFFIXES	MEANING	EXAMPLES
bathy-	deep	**bathy**pnea – To breathe deeply.
-tocia	birth	dys**tocia** – To have a difficult childbirth.
		brady**tocia** – To have a slow childbirth.
hygr-	wet	**hygr**oma – Fluid-filled sac,cyst, or bursa.
		hygrometry – Measurement of moisture in the atmosphere.
-ferous	to bear	lacti**ferous** – To bear or contain milk.
		somni**ferous** – To induce sleep.
pil(o)	hair	e**pil**ation – To remove hair.
		pilosebaceous – Pertaining to a hair follicle and the sebaceous gland.
-agra	seizure; pain	pod**agra** – Pain in the foot caused by gout.
per-	through	**per**cutaneous – Given through or by way of the skin.
		peroral – Given through the mouth.
fiss-	split	**fiss**ure – Any cleft or groove.
		fissula – Small cleft.
-tropia	turn	eso**tropia** – The turning inward of one eye.
		exo**tropia** – The turning outward of one eye.
hemi-	half	**hemi**sphere – Half of a globe or sphere. Also, half of the cerebrum or cerebellum.
		hemiplegia – Paralysis of one half of the body.
pec-	fix; fasten	**pec**tin – Gelatinous polysaccharide that is present in fruits.

MEDICAL ROOTS / PREFIXES / SUFFIXES	MEANING	EXAMPLES
re-	backwards; again	**re**traction – To draw back.
		repeat – To do again.
eu-	good; normal; easy	**eu**pepsia – Good or normal digestion.
		euthanasia – A painless or easy death.
pur(i)	pus	sup**pur**ation – The formation of pus.
		purulent – To be associated with pus.
noct(i)	night	**noct**uria – To urinate frequently during the night.
		noctambulism – Sleepwalking.
acanth(o)	a spine or thorn	**acantho**cyte – An abnormal red blood cell that appears "thorny."
		acantha – A vertebral spinous process.
gelat(o)	freeze; congeal	**gelat**ion – To solidify by cooling.
thec(o)	sheath; case	**thec**a – A case or sheath.
		thecoma – A tumor made up of theca cells.
faci(o)	face	**facio**plasty – Plastic surgery of the face.
		facioplegia – Paralysis of the face.
phleb(o)	vein	**phlebo**stasis – Slow circulation of blood in the veins.
		peri**phleb**itis – Inflammation of the tissues surrounding a vein.
ov(o)	egg	**ov**iduct – A duct that allows the ova or egg to the leave from the ovary and pass to the uterus.
		syn**ov**ia – A fluid that resemble to white of an egg that is secreted by membranes.
nemat-	thread; thin	**nemat**ode – Roundworm.

MEDICAL ROOTS / PREFIXES / SUFFIXES	MEANING	EXAMPLES
ven(o)	vein	**ven**ule – A small vein.
		venostasis – The stoppage of blood flow through the veins.
con-	with; together	**con**nect – To put together.
		contagious – The ability of a disease to be transferred to another.
ton(o)	tone; tension	**tono**metry – The measurement of tension or pressure.
		vaso**ton**ic – Pertaining to the tension or tone of the blood vessels.
bronchiol(o)	bronchiole	**bronchiol**ectasis – Dilation of the bronchioles.
eti(o)	cause	**etio**logy – Study of the cause of disease.
tympan(o)	eardrum	**tympano**centesis – The surgical puncture of the tympanic membrane.
		tympanoplasty – Surgical reconstruction of the tympanic membrane.
alveol(o)	sac	pulmonary **alveo**li – Small sacs at the ends of terminal bronchioles in which respiratory gas exchange occurs.
		dental **alveol**i – The cavities in which the teeth are rooted.
melan(o)	black; melanin	**melano**cyte – A cell which produces melanin or pigment.
		melanonychia – Blackening of the nails.
fus(o)	flow; spindle	dif**fuse** – To pass through or spread widely throughout a tissue or structure.
		fusible – Able to be melted.
pyr(o)	fire; heat; fever	**pyro**gen – A substance which induces a fever.
		pyromania – An obsession with fire.
chlor(o)	green	**chloro**phyll – A green pigment found in plants.
		chloroma – A malignant tumor that is green in color.

MEDICAL ROOTS / PREFIXES / SUFFIXES	MEANING	EXAMPLES
-orrhea	flow; discharge	metr**orrhea** – An abnormal discharge from the uterus.
		galact**orrhea** – Excessive flow of milk.
bry(o)	life	em**bry**o – In humans, the developing organism up to the eighth week.
flagell(o)	whip	**flagell**a – Long, whiplike appendages attached to the surface of a cell that propel the organism.
		flagellation – Whipping one's self for pleasure; the formation of flagella on an organism.
seps(o)	infection	**seps**is – An infection.
lymphangi(o)	lymph vessel	**lymphangi**ectasis – Dilation of a lymph vessel.
		lymphangioma – A tumor made up of forming lymph spaces and channels.
ulcer(o)	ulcer	**ulcer**ation – The development of an ulcer.
		ulcerogenic – Something that causes or leads to ulcers.
stroph(o)	twist	dia**stroph**ic – Bent or curved (e.g. bones).
		strophulus – Papular hives.
anti-	counteractive; against	**anti**dote – An agent or mechanism that counteracts a poison.
		antiemetic – An agent or mechanism that relieves or prevents nausea.
tal(o)	ankle bone; talus	**talo**crural – Pertaining to the talus and the leg bones.
		talofibular – Pertaining to the talus and the fibula.
ile(o)	ileum; the longest portion of the intestine	**ile**ectomy – Surgical excision of the ileum.
		ileitis – Inflammation of the ileum.

MEDICAL ROOTS / PREFIXES / SUFFIXES	MEANING	EXAMPLES
om(o)	shoulder	**om**oclavicular – Pertaining to the shoulder and clavicle.
		omohyoid – Pertaining to the shoulder and the hyoid bone.
myel(o)	bone marrow; spinal cord	**myel**itis – Inflammation of the spinal cord.
		myeloma – A tumor that is made up of bone marrow cells.
bacill-	rod-like	**bacill**us – A genus of rod-shaped bacteria.
		bacilliform – Having a rod-shaped form.
pos(o)	a drink	hyper**pos**ia – Punctuated, irregular increase of fluid ingestion.
		posology – Science or a system of dosage.
test(o)	testicle	**test**algia – Pain of the testicle.
		testosterone – A hormone produced by the testes.
spectr(o)	appearance; that which is seen	**spectr**oscope – Instrument used for revealing and analyzing spectra.
hyp-	beneath; below; under	**hypo**dermic – Below the skin.
		hypoglycemia – An abnormally low blood glucose level.
		hypaxial – Ventral to the long axis of the body.
iso-	equal	**iso**phoria – Equal tension of the vertical muscles in each eye.
		isochromatic – Equal or same color throughout.
agglutin(o)	adhering to one another; clumping	**agglutin**ation – Clumping of cells (often bacteria) after exposure to immunity system agents.
		agglutinin – An antibody which causes its antigen to clump to one another.

MEDICAL ROOTS / PREFIXES / SUFFIXES	MEANING	EXAMPLES
pachy(o)	thick	**pachyo**nychia – Thickening of the nails.
		pachyglossia – Having a thick tongue.
-sis	action	diagno**sis** – Act of diagnosing.
cutane(o)	skin	sub**cutaneo**us – Under the skin.
		per**cutaneo**us – Given through or by way of the skin.
hem(o)	blood	**hem**atemesis – Vomiting blood.
		hemoglobin – A protein found in red blood cells.
flav-	yellow	**flav**in – Water soluble yellow pigments that are diverse in animals and plants.
		***Flav**obacterium* – Genus of gram-negative, aerobic or facultatively anaerobic, soil and water bacteria which are characterized by the yellow pigment they produce.
-mimetic	mimic; copy	sympatho**mimetic** – To mimic the effects caused by stimulation of the sympathetic nervous system.
		radio**mimetic** – Having similar effect to radiation.
appendic(o)	relating or pertaining to an appendix (appendage)	**appendic**olysis – Surgical separation of adhesions from the vermiform appendix.
suf-	under; beneath; below; inferior	**suf**focation – Asphyxiation as by stoppage of respiration.
azot(o)	urea; nitrogen-based waste	**azot**uria – Excessive nitrogen waste in the urine.
		azotemea – Excessive nitrogen waste in the blood.
-pexy	to fasten; fixation	gastro**pexy** – Fixation of the stomach.
		hepato**pexy** – Fixation of the liver to the abdominal wall.

MEDICAL ROOTS / PREFIXES / SUFFIXES	MEANING	EXAMPLES
klept(o)	to steal	**klepto**mania – Compulsive stealing of objects with no personal or monetary value.
lamin(o)	thin layer or sheet; posterior arch of vertebra	**lamin**ated – Arranged in layers.
		laminectomy – Surgical excision of the posterior arch of a vertebra.
caus(o)	burning	**caus**tic – The ability to burn; destroying living tissue.
		causalgia – Burning pain.
ferr(o)	iron	**ferr**odoxin – Nonheme iron-containing protein.
		ferroprotein – Protein combined with an iron-containing radical.
abs-	away from	**abs**cission – Removal by cutting.
		absolute – Free from limitations; unlimited
mes(o)	middle	**meso**derm – The middle germ layer of a forming embryo.
		mesiad – Toward the middle.
cen-	common	**cen**esthesia – The general feeling of the presence of one's own body.
-ptysis	spitting	hemo**ptysis** – To spit up blood.
a(n)-	not; without; away from	**a**febrile – Without fever.
		analgesia – Without pain.
para-	adjacent; beyond	**para**nasal – Adjacent to the nose.
		paranormal – Beyond scientific explanation.
rhag(o)	burst	hemor**rhag**e – The flow of blood out of the vessels; bleeding.
gravid(o)	pregnancy	**gravid**a – A pregnant woman.
		gravidocardiac – Heart disease during pregnancy.

MEDICAL ROOTS / PREFIXES / SUFFIXES	MEANING	EXAMPLES
psychr(o)	cold	**psychro**algia – A painful, cold sensation.
		psychrophilic – Being fond of or liking cold.
man(i)	hand	**mani**pulation – Skillful use of the hands.
duoden(o)	duodenum	**duoden**itis – Inflammation of the duodenum.
		duodenum – The first portion of the small intestine.
sept(o)	wall off; fence	**septo**nasal – Pertaining to the division or wall of the nose.
		septate – To be divided by a septum.
horm(o)	impulse	**horm**one – A chemical impulse sent to affect certain cells or organs.
pept(o)	digestion	**pepto**genic – Something that promotes digestion.
		peptic – Pertaining to digestion.
coll-	glue	**coll**ide – To crash into one another.
		collagen – The major protein component of connective tissue.
irid(o)	iris	**irido**plegia – Paralysis of the sphincter of the iris.
		iridocyclitis – Inflammation of the iris and ciliary body.
-ferent	bear; carry	ef**ferent** – Carrying away from an organ or part.
		de**ferent** – Serving to carry.
-algia	pain	my**algia** – Pain of one or more muscles.
		arthr**algia** – Pain of one or more joints.
picr(o)	bitter	**picr**ic – Extremely bitter.
		picrotoxin – A bitter poison.

MEDICAL ROOTS / PREFIXES / SUFFIXES	MEANING	EXAMPLES
pag(o)	fix	thoraco**pag**us – Conjoined twins connected in or near the sternal region.
natr(o)	salt; sodium	**natri**uresis – Excretion of sodium in the urine.
		hyper**natr**emia – An elevated amount of sodium in the blood.
spher(o)	round; sphere-like	hemi**spher**e – Half of a globe or sphere. Also, half of the cerebrum or cerebellum.
		spherocyte – A sphere-shaped cell.
teg(u)	cover	in**teg**ument – Covering.
-philia	like; affinity for	hydro**philia** – Having an affinity for water.
		necro**philia** – having a sexual attraction to dead bodies.
nom(i)	law; custom	taxo**nom**y – The orderly classification of organisms into appropriate groupings.
-clast	break	osteo**clast** – A cell that breaks down bone.
		icono**clast** – A person who seeks to break or destroy popular ideas.
squam(o)	scale; skin	de**squam**ation – The shedding or peeling of skin.
		squamous – Scaly.
papill(o)	nipple-like; optic disk	**papillo**ma – A small, benign epithelial tumor; wart.
		papillitis – Inflammation of the optic disk.
thorac(o)	chest	**thorac**algia – Chest pain.
		thoracostenosis – An abnormal contraction of the thorax.
cement(o)	cement	**cement**um – The bone-like covering of the root of the tooth.
scirrh(o)	hard	**scirrho**us – Pertaining to hardness.

MEDICAL ROOTS / PREFIXES / SUFFIXES	MEANING	EXAMPLES
rect(o)	rectum; straight	**recto**cele – Herniation of the rectum into the vagina.
		rectification – To make straight or correct.
-phoria	mood; feeling	eu**phoria** – To be happy; content.
		dys**phoria** – Not satisfied; impatient.
scat(o)	dung	**scat**ology – Diagnostic study and analysis of feces.
hered(i)	heir	**hered**itary – Genetically passed from parent to child.
semin(o)	semen; seed	**semin**uria – The presence of semen in the urine.
		in**semin**ation – To inject semen into the reproductive tract of a female.
glyc(o)	sugar	**glyco**lysis – The breakdown of glucose.
		hyper**glyc**emia – Elevated blood sugar level.
kary(o)	nucleus	**karyo**rrhexis – Rupture of the cell nucleus.
		karyokinesis – Division of the cell nucleus.
pyl(e)	door	**pyl**ephlebitis – Inflammation of the portal vein.
hyal(o)	glass-like	**hyal**ine – Glassy or translucent.
		hyaloplasm – A glass-like fluid found in the cell.
sym-	with; together	**sym**pathomimetic – To mimic the effects caused by stimulation of the sympathetic nervous system.
		symphysis – To grow together.
trip(o)	rub	litho**trip**sy – Destruction of a calcium stone within the urinary system or gallbladder and washing away of the particles.

MEDICAL ROOTS / PREFIXES / SUFFIXES	MEANING	EXAMPLES
-pnea	breath; respiration	ortho**pnea** – Difficulty breathing unless one is in the upright position.
		dys**pnea** – Difficulty breathing.
areola	a small area	**areola –** The small circular area of different pigment that surrounds the nipple of the breast.
		Chaussier's **areola** – The inflamed area immediately around a cancerous pustule.
derm(o)	skin	**derm**atology – A branch of medicine that deals with the skin.
		erythro**derm**a – An abnormal redness of the skin.
tibi(o)	tibia	**tibio**femoral – Pertaining to the tibia and femur.
		tibiofibular – Pertaining to the tibia and fibula.
myc(o)	fungus	dermato**myco**sis – A fungal infection of the skin.
		onycho**myco**sis – A fungal infection of the nails.
cardi(o)	heart	**cardio**megaly – Abnormal enlargement of the heart.
		cardiology – Study of the heart.
ser(o)	serum; watery substance	**sero**purulent – To be both serous and purulent.
		serosanguineous – Made up of both serum and blood.
cell(o)	room; cell	**cell**ular – Pertaining to or made of cells; consisting of small compartments.
-osis	process; disorder; disease	dyshidr**osis** – A disorder of the sweat glands.
		dermat**osis** – A disease of the skin.
dif-	apart; not	**dif**ficult – Not easy.
		diffraction – The spreading apart of light.

MEDICAL ROOTS / PREFIXES / SUFFIXES	MEANING	EXAMPLES
pre-	before	**pre**natal – Happening before birth.
		preterm – Happening before completion of the full term.
col(o)	large intestine	**col**itis – Inflammation of the colon.
		colic – Abdominal pain.
peri-	around	**peri**phery – The outward surface of a body.
		perimeter – The border or boundary of an area.
ac-	to; add	**ac**cumulation – To add onto or build up.
		accustom – To become familiar with.
estr(o)	female	**estro**gen – A female hormone.
dys-	bad; improper; difficult	**dys**function – Not working correctly.
		dyslexia – The inability to read, spell, and write words correctly.
ankyl(o)	crooked; fixed	**ankylo**sis – Inability of a joint to move.
		ankylosing spondylitis – A disease resulting in a severe immobility of the spine.
plumb(o)	lead	**plumb**ic – Pertaining to or associated with lead.
		plumbism – Lead poisoning.
-malacia	softening	osteo**malacia** – Softening of the bone.
		encephalo**malacia** – Softening of the brain.
cari(o)	putrescence	**cari**es – Decay of bone or teeth.
		cariogenesis – The development of bone or tooth decay.

MEDICAL ROOTS / PREFIXES / SUFFIXES	MEANING	EXAMPLES
pulmon(o)	lung	**pulmon**ary – Associated with the lungs.
		pulmonectomy – Surgical excision of a lung.
oste(o)	bone	**osteo**blast – A cell from which bone develops.
		osteomalacia – Softening of the bone.
chondr(o)	cartilage	**chondro**blast – A cell that produces cartilage that is in the early stages of growth.
		chondropathy – Disease of the cartilage.
quasi-	as though	**quasi**dominance – Mimicking of dominance in inheritance caused by mating a carrier of a recessive gene with an individual homozygous for the gene.
vulv(o)	vulva	**vulv**ectomy – Surgical excision of the vulva.
		vulvitis – Inflammation of the vulva.
ole(o)	oil	**ole**aginous – To be oily or greasy.
		olearthrosis – Injection of oil into a joint.
psych(o)	mind	**psycho**logist – Someone who studies the mind.
		psychopathy – Any mental disorder.
circu-	around	**circu**mcision – Removal of the skin that wraps around the tip of the penis.
		circulation – Movement of blood throughout the body.
-phoresis	support; bear; carry	electro**phoresis** – Transmission of electrical current.
		dia**phoresis** – Perspiration; secretion of sweat.
ef-	out of; from	**ef**ferent – Going away from an organ or part.
		effusion – The escape of fluid; pouring out of.

MEDICAL ROOTS / PREFIXES / SUFFIXES	MEANING	EXAMPLES
staphyl(o)	cluster of grapes; uvula	**staphylo**coccus – A round shaped gram-positive bacteria that is usually found in clusters like grapes.
		staphyline – Pertaining to the uvula.
rhaph(o)	suture	arterior**rhaph**y – Suture of an artery.
dolor(o)	pain	**dolor**imeter – An instrument for measuring pain.
		dolorology – The study of pain.
acar(o)	mite	**acaro**dermatitis – A skin inflammation that is caused by mites.
		acarology – The study of mites and ticks.
vas(o)	vessel	**vaso**tonic – Pertaining to the tension or tone of the blood vessels.
		vasodilation – Dilation of the blood vessels.
cer(o)	wax	**cer**oplasty – Making anatomical models in wax.
		cerumen – Earwax.
-ole	small; little	arteri**ole** – A small artery.
		bronchi**ole** – A small extension of a bronchus.
brady-	slow	**brady**cardia – Slowing of the heart rate.
		bradypnea – Abnormal slowness of breath.
-partum	birth	post-**partum** – Occurring after birth.
ophthalm(o)	eye	ex**ophthalmo**s – Protrusion of the eyeball.
		ophthalmorrhea – Bleeding from the eye.
cili-	eyelids	**cili**ary – Associated with or pertaining to the eye and its surrounding structures.
		ciliectomy – Surgical excision of part of the eyelid.

MEDICAL ROOTS / PREFIXES / SUFFIXES	MEANING	EXAMPLES
-ous	pertaining or referring to; full of; abounding	aque**ous** – Full of water.
		frivol**ous** – Very carefree; not serious.
flu(x)	flow	**flu**id – A liquid or gas.
		de**flux**ion – Sudden disappearance; copious discharge; falling out (e.g. hair).
antero-	in front of	**antero**grade – Moving or extending forward.
		anterolateral – A direction toward or location in the front and to one side.
-cyte	cell	leuko**cyte** – White blood cell.
		erythro**cyte** – Red blood cell.
dactyl(o)	digit	campto**dactyl**y – Having a permanently bent finger.
		hexa**dactyl**y – Having six fingers or toes on a hand or foot.
gymn(o)	naked	**gymn**osperm – Seed that is unprotected by ovary or fruit.
-orrhagia	profuse bleeding	omphal**orrhagia** – Bleeding of the navel.
		men**orrhagia** – Profuse bleeding from the uterus.
ob-	against	**ob**tusion – Deadening of sensitiveness.
		obstruction – A blockage.
igni(o)	fire	**igni**te – To light on fire.
		ignipuncture – Puncture of the body using hot instruments for therapeutic purposes.
-pheresis	remove	plasma**pheresis** – To remove plasma from the blood.
chromat(o)	color	poly**chromat**ic – Having many colors.
		chromaturia – Abnormal urine color.

MEDICAL ROOTS / PREFIXES / SUFFIXES	MEANING	EXAMPLES
supra-	above; over	**supra**spinal – Above the spine.
		supracostal – Above the ribs.
ter-	thrice	**ter**nary – Third; made of three chemicals.
		tertian – Recurring every third day.
micr(o)	small	**micro**scopic – Too small to be seen with the unaided eye.
		microstomia – An unusually small mouth.
adenoid(o)	similar to a gland	**adenoid**ectomy – Surgical excision of the adenoids, lymphoid tissue located in the pharynx.
		adenoiditis – Inflammation of the adenoids.
my(o)	muscle	**myo**globin – A protein found in the muscle.
		myasthenia – Muscular weakness (e.g. myasthenia gravis).
trache(o)	trachea	**tracheo**tomy – Surgical incision of the trachea through the neck.
		tracheocele – A herniation of the tracheal mucous membrane.
centr-	center	**centr**iciput – The center portion of the upper surface of the head.
		centripetal – Toward a center.
pseud(o)	fake; false	**pseudo**cyesis – A false pregnancy.
		pseudopod – A false foot.
-centesis	puncture	amnio**centesis** – The surgical procedure of inserting a needle through the abdominal wall and uterus to obtain amniotic fluid for tests.
		entero**centesis** – Surgical puncture of the intestine to withdraw gas or fluid.

MEDICAL ROOTS / PREFIXES / SUFFIXES	MEANING	EXAMPLES
herni(o)	hernia; rupture	**herni**ated – To stick out abnormally.
		hernioplasty – Surgery to repair a hernia.
ren(o)	kidney	**ren**in – An enzyme of the kidney.
		renoprival – Pertaining to a lack of kidney function.
acu(o)	sharpness, often related to sight or sound	**acu**ity – Pertaining to clarity.
		acupuncture – A mechanism to relieve pain by inserting needles in specific areas of the body.
-crasia	mixture	dys**crasia** – An abnormal mixture of the blood.
gemin-	twin	**gemin**ate – Paired.
		geminal – Substituent atoms or groups attached to the same atom in a molecule.
crani(o)	skull	**cranio**tomy – Surgery in which the skull is opened.
		craniomalacia – Unusual softening of the skull.
-pepsia	digestion	eu**pepsia** – Good or normal digestion.
		dys**pepsia** – Difficult digestion.
nebul(o)	cloud; fog; mist	**nebul**a – A cloudy spot on the cornea.
		nebulize – To make into a mist.
-ectasia	dilation; expansion	tangi**ectasia** – Dark red blotches on the skin that are caused by abnormal dilation of groups of capillaries.
		col**ectasia** – Dilation of the colon.
corpor-	body	**corpor**ation – A group of people that act as one body.

MEDICAL ROOTS / PREFIXES / SUFFIXES	MEANING	EXAMPLES
desm(o)	ligament	**desmo**plasia – Formation of a ligament.
		desmotomy – Surgical incision of a ligament.
-cept	receive	inter**cept** – Prevent someone or something from continuing to its destination.
		re**cept**or – A region of tissue, or a molecule on a cell surface, that responds specifically to a certain neurotransmitter, hormone, antigen, or other substance.
phot(o)	light	**photo**phobia – The fear of light.
		photodermatitis – Inflammation of the skin caused by exposure to sunlight.
ischi(o)	hip; haunch; ischium	**ischio**dynia – Pain in the ischium.
		ischiorectal – Pertaining to the ischium and rectum.
-ol	oil	choleste**rol** – Sterol precursor of bile acids and steroid hormones and a component of cell membranes.
ana-	upward; backward, again, excessive	**ana**bolism – A building process where simple substances are converted to more complex compounds.
		anaplasia – Cells begin to grow in a more primitive pattern.
-cyesis	pregnancy	pseudo**cyesis** – A false pregnancy
plic(o)	fold	**plic**ate – To fold into pleats.
		plication – An operation in which a structure is folded or tucked in order to shorten it.
mne-	pertaining to memory	a**mne**sia – Memory loss.
		mnemonic – Special technique used to improve memory.
eryth-	red	**eryth**ematous – Redness of the skin, inflammation.

MEDICAL ROOTS / PREFIXES / SUFFIXES	MEANING	EXAMPLES
taut(o)	same	**taut**omerism – Relationship between two constitutional isomers in equilibrium that can freely change from one to the other.
lord(o)	bent; curved	**lordo**sis – A curving of the spine.
ir-	not; within	**ir**rational – Not rational.
		irradiation – To expose to radiation; to put rays into.
-stringent	tighten; draw tight	a**stringent** – Causing contraction.
-ary	pertaining to or associated with	pulmon**ary** – Associated with the lungs.
		integument**ary** – Associated with the integument (the skin).
dis-	apart; not	**dis**locate – To take apart or put out of place.
		disability – Not able to function normally.
gonad(o)	reproductive glands	**gonado**toxic – Having a harmful effect of the gonads.
		gonadectomy – Surgical removal of an ovary or testis.
im-	not; within	**im**mature – Not fully developed.
		immersion – To dip something into a liquid.
scler(o)	hard	**sclero**derma – A hardening of the skin.
		sclerosis – The hardening of tissue.
mal-	bad	**mal**evolent – To wish evil on someone.
		malformation – A bad or faulty formation.
sacchar-	sugar	**sacchar**ide – Among a group of carbohydrates, including the sugars.
		saccharin – Crystalline compound several hundred times sweeter than sucrose.

MEDICAL ROOTS / PREFIXES / SUFFIXES	MEANING	EXAMPLES
blephar(o)	eyelid	**blepharo**tomy – Surgical incision of the eyelid.
		blepharitis – Inflammation of the eyelid.
patell(o)	kneecap	**patell**ectomy – Surgical excision of the kneecap.
		patella – Kneecap.
hipp(o)	horse	**hipp**ocampus – Curved elevation in the floor of the inferior horn of the lateral ventricle.
		hippodrome – Arena set apart for horse and chariot races.
super-	above; beyond; in excess	**super**motility – More motility than normal.
		supernutrition – An excess of nutrition.
gli(o)	glue	neuro**gli**a – A type of cells in the brain and spinal cord that provide support for neurons.
		glioma – A tumor composed of neuroglia.
gen(i)	chin	**geni**culum – Anatomical nomenclature for a sharp bend in a small structure or organ.
acoust(o)	pertaining or relating to the perception of sound	**acousto**gram – A graph of the curves of sound.
		external **acoust**ic meatus – The external passage to the middle ear.
periton(e)	peritoneum	**peritone**algia – Pain in the peritoneum.
		peritonitis – Inflammation of the peritoneum.
vert(i)	turn	in**vert** – Upside down or in the opposite position.
lapar(o)	flank; loin; abdomen	**laparo**tomy – Surgical incision of the abdomen.
		laparoscopy – The use of a laparoscope to examine the inside of the abdomen.

MEDICAL ROOTS / PREFIXES / SUFFIXES	MEANING	EXAMPLES
rhe(o)	flow	diar**rhe**a – Frequent evacuation of watery feces.
-para	birth	nulli**para** – A woman who has never given birth to a child.
		primi**para** – A woman who is pregnant for the first time.
sect(i)	cut	bi**sect** – Cut into two parts.
		dis**sect** – Cut apart; expose structures on a cadaver for study.
erot(o)	relating to or associated with sexual desire	**eroto**phobia – Fear of sexual desire.
		erotism – One's sexual desire.
orch(o)	testes	**orch**iopathy – A disease of the testes.
		orchiotomy – Surgical incision into a testis.
femor(o)	femur	**femor**ocele – Femoral hernia.
-ule	small; little	ven**ule** – A small vein.
		cell**ule** – A small cell.
in-	not; within	**in**adequate – Not adequate.
		incision – To cut into.
pluri-	more	**pluri**glandular – Pertaining to several glands.
		pluripotency – Ability to develop in one of several ways or to affect several organs or tissues.
axi(o)	axis	ab**axi**al – Away from the axis of a structure or part.
xanth(o)	yellow	**xantho**derma – A yellowish discoloration of the skin.
		xanthochromic – To have a yellow discoloration.

MEDICAL ROOTS / PREFIXES / SUFFIXES	MEANING	EXAMPLES
argyr(o)	silver	**argyr**ia – Silver poisoning.
		argyrophil – Able to bind silver.
holo-	entire	**holo**enzyme – The entire enzyme composed of the coenzyme and apoenzyme.
tonsill(o)	tonsils	**tonsill**itis – Inflammation of the tonsils.
		tonsillectomy – Surgical excision of a tonsil.
exo-	outside	**exo**skeleton – An outer covering.
		exocrine – Secretion of hormones outside via a duct.
pharmac(o)	drug	**pharmaco**logy – The study of drugs.
		pharmacognosy – The study of natural drugs.
mechan(o)	machine	**mechan**oreceptor – A receptor that responds to mechanical pressures or distortions.
-fect	make	af**fect** – A show of emotion; to produce an effect.
		in**fect**ious – Caused by or capable of being transmitted by an infection.
colp(o)	vagina	**colp**algia – Pain in the vagina.
		colpohyperplasia – Excessive thickening of the wall of the vagina.
-pathy	disease	orchio**pathy** – A disease of the testes.
		hystero**pathy** – A disease of the uterus.
-form	shape	uni**form** – Having the same shape.
-logy	study of	immuno**logy** – The study of the immune system.
		nephro**logy** – The study of the kidneys.

MEDICAL ROOTS / PREFIXES / SUFFIXES	MEANING	EXAMPLES
vagin(o)	vagina	**vagino**dynia – Pain in the vagina.
		vaginitis – Inflammation of the vagina.
-salpinx	fallopian tube	pyo**salpinx** – The accumulation of pus in a fallopian tube.
-ac	pertaining or referring to	cardi**ac** – Relating to the heart.
		mani**ac** – An individual who experiences mania.
spondyl(o)	vertebrae	**spondylo**pyosis – The formation of pus on a vertebra.
		spondylolysis – The breaking down of a vertebra.
meta-	after; beyond; change	**meta**basis – The change in course of a disease.
		metapneumonic – To follow pneumonia.
flect(o)	bend	de**flect**ion – Deviation from a straight line.
		in**flect**ion – The act or state of bending inward.
prurit(o)	itch	**prurit**us – To itch.
eury-	wide	**eury**cephalic – Having a wide head.
		euryon – A point on the parietal bone of the skull marking the greatest transverse diameter of the skull.
-graph	record; write	calli**graph**er – Fancy writing.
		baro**graph** – An instrument that records the atmospheric pressure.
steat(o)	fat	**steato**rrhea – An excess of fat in the feces.
		steatonecrosis – The death of fatty tissue.
-oid	resembling; like; equivalent	lip**oid** – To resemble fat.
		choan**oid** – Funnel-shaped.

MEDICAL ROOTS / PREFIXES / SUFFIXES	MEANING	EXAMPLES
noto-	pertaining to the back	**noto**chord – A rod-shaped system of cells on the dorsal aspect of an embryo serving, as the center for the development of the skeletal system.
sial(o)	saliva	**sial**ectasia – The dilation of a salivary duct.
		sialagogue – An agent that stimulates the flow of saliva.
helc(o)	sore; ulcer	kerato**helc**osis – Ulcer of the cornea.
-cele	hernia; tumor; hollow	myo**cele** – Protrusion of muscle.
		aero**cele** – An air-filled pouch, particularly one attached to the trachea or larynx.
plex(o)	network; braid	**plex**us – A network or intertangling of nerves.
		plexiform – Resembling a plexus.
-emia	blood	an**emia** – Lack of red blood cells.
		septic**emia** – Pathogenic bacteria in the bloodstream; blood poisoning.
-facient	make	cale**facient** – That which causes warmth.
		aborti**facient** – That which causes a miscarriage.
-stasis	to stop; stagnation	hemo**stasis** – The stoppage of blood flow.
		chole**stasis** – The stoppage of bile flow.
ad-	to; add	**ad**duct – Movement toward the midline of a structure. To adduct the arm is to bring it down the side of the body. To adduct the fingers is to bring them together so they are closer to the midline of the upper extremity.
		caud**ad** – Toward the cauda (tail). In the human, this corresponds with the coccyx bone at the distal inferior end of the vertebral column.

MEDICAL ROOTS / PREFIXES / SUFFIXES	MEANING	EXAMPLES
episi(o)	pubic region	**episi**ostenosis – Narrowing of the vulvar orifice.
		episiotomy – An incision made into the perineum and vagina to prevent tearing during delivery.
sangui-	blood	**sangui**facient – Pertaining to the formation of red blood cells.
		sanguinopurulent – Containing both blood and pus.
the(o)	put; place	syn**the**sis – Combining simpler parts to create a whole.
phyt(o)	plant	spermato**phyt**e – A group of plants that bear seeds.
		dermato**phyt**e – Fungus of the skin; a "skin plant".
balan(o)	pertaining or referring to the glans penis	**balano**plasty – Surgical repair of the glans penis.
		balanitis – Inflammation of the glans penis.
eso-	inside; within	**eso**tropia – Cross-eyed; when one eye turns inward towards the other eye.
audi(o)	hearing	**audio**logy – The science of hearing.
		auditory – Pertaining or related to the ear or the perception of sound.
-sclerosis	hardening	arterio**sclerosis** – Hardening of the arteries.
		arteriolo**sclerosis** – Hardening of arterioles.
-megaly	enlarged	acro**megaly** – Enlargement of the extremities of the body (fingers, nose, jaw) by excessive growth hormone.
		cephalo**megaly** – Enlargement of the head.
trans-	through; across	**trans**lucent – Allowing light to pass through.
		transfusion – The process of introducing whole blood into the bloodstream.
epipl(o)	omentum	**epipl**oic – Pertaining to the omentum.

MEDICAL ROOTS / PREFIXES / SUFFIXES	MEANING	EXAMPLES
albin(o)	white	**albin**uria – Having white or pale urine.
		albinism – Not having normal pigmentation in the body.
-thorax	chest	hemo**thorax** – The presence of blood in the chest.
		pneumo**thorax** – The presence of air or gas in the chest.
nymph(o)	bride	**nymph**otomy – Surgical excision of the nymphae (i.e. clitoris).
or(o)	mouth	intra**or**al – Within the mouth.
		oral – Pertaining to the mouth.
hydr(o)	water	**hydr**ation – To combine or supply with water.
		hydrophobic – Not absorbing water.
genit(o)	referring to birth	**genit**alia – The reproductive organs, more often referring to those that are external.
		genitourinary – Pertaining to the genital and urinary systems.
lys(o)	breakdown; split; dissolution	lipo**lys**is – The breakdown of fat.
		hydro**lys**is – The splitting of water molecules.
palat(o)	palate	**palato**plegia – Paralysis of the palate.
		palatitis – Inflammation of the tongue.
adren(o)	pertaining or referring to the adrenal gland	**adren**alin – A name for epinephrine, a hormone secreted by cells of the medulla of the adrenal gland.
		adrenomegaly – An increase in size of an adrenal gland.
gest(o)	bear; carry	in**gest**ant – Substance that is taken into the body by mouth or through the digestive system.

MEDICAL ROOTS / PREFIXES / SUFFIXES	MEANING	EXAMPLES
tax(o)	order; arrangement	a**tax**ia – Having no coordination.
		taxonomy – The grouping of organisms according to shared characteristics.
laryng(o)	larynx	**laryngo**plegia – Paralysis of the larynx.
		laryngostenosis – A narrowing of the larynx.
ba(o)	walk; stand	a**ba**sia – Inability to walk.
isch(o)	suppress	**isch**emia – A decrease in blood supply.
		ischuria – A decrease in urine flow.
opac(o)	not translucent; dark	**opac**ity – The state of being opaque or impervious to light.
cerebell(o)	cerebellum	**cerebell**ar – Associated with or pertaining to the cerebellum.
		cerebellitis – Inflammation of the cerebellum.
phall-	penis	**phall**oplasty – Plastic surgery of the penis.
		phallitis – Inflammation of the penis.
-genesis	origin; generation	carcino**genesis** – The growth of cancer.
		oo**genesis** – The development of the ova.
osm(o)	smell; odor; impulse	an**osm**ia – Not having the ability to smell.
		osmophobia – The fear of odors or smells.
		osmoregulation – The maintenance of internal osmotic pressure in relation to the surrounding medium.
tachy-	swift; rapid; fast	**tachy**cardia – A rapid heart rate.
		tachyphagia – To eat rapidly.

MEDICAL ROOTS / PREFIXES / SUFFIXES	MEANING	EXAMPLES
porphyr(o)	purple	**porphyr**inuria – A condition in which the urine is purple.
ec-	out of; outside	**ec**centric – Outside of the norm; a person who acts outside of normal character.
		ectopic – Not in the normal position.
albumin(o)	pertaining or referring to a protein	**albumin** – A soluble protein.
		albuminocholia – Protein in the bile.
prot(o)	first	**proto**duodenum – The first part of the duodenum.
		protopathic – The part that senses pain or is affected first.
choledoch(o)	common bile duct	**choledoch**al – Pertaining to the common bile duct.
		choledochitis – Inflammation of the common bile duct.
ret-	network	**ret**icular – Resembling a net.
		reticulocyte – A red blood cell that contains a network.
crur(o)	shin, leg	**crur**al – Pertaining to or resembling a lower limb.
		talo**crur**al – Pertaining to the talus and the leg bones.
odyn(o)	pain	gastr**odyn**ia – Pain in the stomach.
		odynophagia – Pain when swallowing.
arcus	bow; arch	**arcus** sinilis – A gray line of lipid degradation surrounding the margin of the cornea.
orb(i)	circle	**orb**icular – Circular; rounded.
		orbit – The bony cavity containing the eye and its vessels, nerves, and muscles.
carcin(o)	cancer	**carcino**gen – A substance that causes cancer.
		carcinoma – A cancerous tumor.

MEDICAL ROOTS / PREFIXES / SUFFIXES	MEANING	EXAMPLES
uln(o)	ulna; elbow	**uln**ar – Pertaining to the ulna.
		ulnoradial – Pertaining the ulna and radius.
neutr(o)	neutral; neither	**neutro**n – A particle that has no charge.
		neutrophil – A cell that can be stained by neutral dyes.
-id	form; resemblance	lipo**id** – To resemble fat.
		plast**id** – Any of a class of small organelles in the cytoplasm of plant cells, containing pigment or food.
-cusis	hearing	ana**cusis** – Completely deaf.
		presby**cusis** – The loss of hearing the comes with old age.
pleur(o)	rib; side	**pleur**a – A membrane surrounding the lungs.
		pleurocentesis – To remove fluid from the lungs by puncturing the pleural cavity.
-ism	a suffix which makes the word a noun	alcohol**ism** – Disorder marked by alcohol abuse.
		isomer**ism** – Two compounds with the same number of atoms of each element, but in different arrangement.
top(o)	place	**top**esthesia – The ability to recognize the sensation of touch.
		topography – The description of a particular part of the body.
choan(o)	funnel	**choano**id – Funnel-shaped.
		choana – An opening into the nasopharynx of the nasal cavity.
ball(o)	throw	**ball**ismus – Jerking of the limbs.
entom(o)	insect	**entom**ology – Study of insects.
		entomophthorales – An order of fungi that typically parasitically infects insects.

MEDICAL ROOTS / PREFIXES / SUFFIXES	MEANING	EXAMPLES
-capnia	carbon dioxide	hyper**capnia** – Excessive amounts of carbon dioxide in the lungs.
salping(o)	uterine tube	**salpingo**cele – Herniation of the uterine tube.
		salpingectomy – Surgical excision of the uterine tube.
ment(o)	mind; chin	**mento**labial – Associated with or pertaining to the chin and lip.
		mentoplasty – Plastic surgery on the chin.
-penia	decrease; deficiency	erythro**penia** – A low number of red blood cells.
		leuko**penia** – A low number of white blood cells.
gland(o)	acorn	**gland**ular – Pertaining or similar to a gland.
algesi(o)	perception of pain	**analgesi**a – Without pain.
		analgesic – An agent that relieves pain.
pharyng(o)	throat; pharynx	**pharyngo**cele – A hernia of the pharynx.
		pharyngomycosis – A fungal infection of the pharynx.
odont(o)	tooth	ortho**dont**ics – A branch of dentistry dealing with the correction of teeth.
		odontalgia – A toothache.
flex(o)	bend	re**flex** – Action or movement brought on by the automatic response of the nervous system.
		flexion – The act or condition of bending.
condyl(o)	rounded projection	**condyl**e – A rounded projection on the bone.
		condyloma – A growth on the skin.
omphal(o)	navel	**omphalo**rrhagia – Bleeding of the navel.
		omphalotomy – The cutting of the umbilical cord.

MEDICAL ROOTS / PREFIXES / SUFFIXES	MEANING	EXAMPLES
cret(o)	distinguish; separate; growth	ac**cret**ion – Growth by accumulation.
		dis**cret**e – Made up of separate parts.
ex-	out of; away	**ex**cavation – To hollow out.
		excise – To take out by cutting.
rhex(i)	burst	metro**rhex**is – Rupture of the uterus.
luc(o)	light; shine; transparent	trans**luc**ent – Allowing light to pass through.
		lucent – Clear; shining.
cephal(o)	head	**cephalo**pod – A mollusk belonging to the class cephalopoda, which are defined by having tentacles attached to a large head.
		cephalomegaly – Enlargement of the head.
nod(o)	knot	**nod**osity – A node or having nodes.
mandibul(o)	mandible	**mandibul**a – The mandible.
		mandibular – Associated with or pertaining to the mandible.
punct(i)	pierce	**punct**ate – Spotted as marked with points or punctures.
		punctiform – Pointed.
gloss(o)	tongue	**gloss**ectomy – Surgical excision of all or a portion of the tongue.
		glossotrichia – A hairy tongue.
dur(o)	hard	in**dur**ation – Hardening; In medicine, an area of the body that has hardened.
		dura mater – The tough, outermost membrane of the brain.

MEDICAL ROOTS / PREFIXES / SUFFIXES	MEANING	EXAMPLES
pleth(o)	fill	**pleth**ora – Excess of blood.
		plethysmograph – Instrument used for recording variations in volume of an organ, part, or limb.
an(o)	anus	**ano**sigmoidoscopy – A procedure in which an endoscope is advanced through the anus to examine the rectum and sigmoid colon.
		anovaginal – Associated with the anus and vagina.
mort(o)	fatal; death	**mort**al – Pertaining to death; deadly.
		im**mort**ality – Having a life that is unending.
glomerul(o)	little ball	**glomerul**us – A small cluster (e.g. blood vessels or nerve fibers).
-esis	act; process	gen**esis** – The act or process of originating or giving birth.
		cytokin**esis** – Final stage of cell division when the cytoplasm splits.
-paresis	partial paralysis	hemi**paresis** – Partial paralysis of one half of the body.
		gastro**paresis** – A partial paralysis of the stomach.
bucc(o)	cheek	**bucc**a – The cheek.
gangli(o)	ganglion; swelling; knot	**ganglio**nitis – Inflammation of a ganglion.
		ganglionectomy – Surgical excision of a ganglion.
-ode	road, path, resemblance	cath**ode** – The electric node to which positive charge is attracted.
		nemat**ode** – Roundworm.
homo-	like; same	**homo**type – One part having reversed symmetry with its pair (e.g. hands).
		homogenous – Made up of the same substances or parts.
strict(o)	tighten; draw tight	con**strict**ion – Narrowing or compression of a part.

MEDICAL ROOTS / PREFIXES / SUFFIXES	MEANING	EXAMPLES
idi(o)	distinct; separate; peculiar; self	**idio**pathic – Having no known cause.
		idiomorphic – Having a distinct form.
path(o)	disease	**patho**logical – Related to pathology (disease).
		pathogenesis – The development of a disease.
erg(o)	work	**ergo**nomics – The study of humans in the workplace.
		ex**ergo**nic – The release of energy.
as-	to, when preceding the consonant *s*	**as**similate – take in and understand; absorb and digest.
bas-	base	**bas**ophil – Readily stained with basic dyes.
		basilad – Toward the base.
mamm(o)	breast	**mammo**gram – An x-ray of the breast.
		sub**mamm**ary – Below the breast.
ambi-	both; around	**ambi**dextrous – Can use either hand well.
		ambient temperature – The surrounding temperature.
mono-	only; single; solo	**mono**cular – Having only one eye.
		monochromatic – Having only one color.
-crine	secrete	endo**crine** – Secretion of hormones internally into the blood.
		exo**crine** – Secretion of hormones externally into a duct.
phac(o)	lens	**phaco**cele – Hernia of the eye lens.
		phacomalacia – Softening of the eye lens.

MEDICAL ROOTS / PREFIXES / SUFFIXES	MEANING	EXAMPLES
brachi(o)	arm	**brachi**al – Pertaining to the arm.
		brachialgia – Pain in the arm.
phon(o)	sound	**phono**asthenia – Weakness of voice.
		phonosurgery – Surgery to enhance the voice.
cyan(o)	blue	**cyano**bacteria – Blue-green algae.
		cyanopsia – A problem with the eye that causes things to appear blue.
-phragm	wall; fence; stop up	dia**phragm** – A wall that separates two cavities in the body.
astr(o)	star	**astro**cyte – A star-shaped cell of the central nervous system which has an ectodermal origin.
		astrocytoma – A tumor of astrocytes.
ede-	swelling	**ede**ma – Swelling due to build up of fluid.
		edemagen – Something that causes edema.
-crescence	growth	ex**crescence** – Anything growing out unnaturally from anything else such as a wart or tumor.
		con**crescence** – Growing together of parts that were orignially separate.
sapr(o)	decay	**sapro**be – An organism that feeds on decaying matter.
		saprozoic – To live on decaying matter.
oophor(o)	ovary	**oophor**ectomy – Surgical removal of one or both ovaries.
		oophorocystosis – The formation of ovarian cysts.

MEDICAL ROOTS / PREFIXES / SUFFIXES	MEANING	EXAMPLES
com-	with; together	**com**mensalism – A relationship between two organisms in which one benefits while the other is unaffected.
		compound – Made up of two or more parts.
heter(o)	other; different	**hetero**geneous – Made of different substances; not alike.
		heterocrine – Secreting more than one substance or matter.
scoli(o)	bent; crooked	**scolio**sis – A curving of the spine.
		scoliosiometry – The measurement of the curvature of the spine.
tect(i)	cover	pro**tect**in – Membrane-bound protein that prevents insertion of the membrane attack complex into the membrane.
later(o)	to the side	ventro**later**al – Pertaining to the front and side.
		lateroversion – A turning to one side.
append(o)	relating or pertaining to an appendix (appendage)	**append**ectomy – Surgical excision of the vermiform appendix.
gust(o)	taste	**gust**atory – Pertaining to or associated with taste.
		gustin – A polypeptide present in saliva.
terat(o)	monster	**terato**ma – A tumor that is made up of different types of tissue.
		teratogen – An agent that causes abnormal prenatal development.
mani-	mental aberration	**mani**ac – Individual exhibiting characteristics of extreme or wild behavior.
lumin(o)	light; cavity inside a tubular structure	**lumin**escence – To give off light without heat.
		luminal – Associated with or pertaining to a cavity in a tubular organ.

MEDICAL ROOTS / PREFIXES / SUFFIXES	MEANING	EXAMPLES
pleo-	more	**pleo**morphic – Existing in more than one form.
		pleocytosis – Having more than the normal number of cells in cerebrospinal fluid.
hamart(o)	fault	**hamart**oma – Benign tumor-like nodule in which cells normally present are disorderly and out of proportion.
glott(o)	tongue; language	**glott**is – Vocal apparatus of the larnyx.
		glottography – Record of the movements of the vocal cords.
nev(o)	mole	**nev**olipoma – Nevus with a large amount of fibrofatty tissue.
		nevus – Birthmark; congenital skin lesion; hamartoma consisting of a stable, circumscribed, malformation of the skin.
arachn(o)	spider	**arachno**id – Similar to a spider web. The arachnoid is the membrane between the pia mater and dura mater; all three form the meninges, which surrounds the brain.
		arachnodactyly – Unusually long and thin fingers and toes.
hypn(o)	sleep	**hypno**sis – To put someone in a sleep-like state.
		hypnalgia – Pain during sleep.
spers(i)	scatter	a**sperse** – To sprinkle water or dust.
		di**sperse** – To scatter parts (e.g. parts of a tumor).
post-	after; behind	**post**partum – Occurring after birth.
		postmortem – Occurring after death.
ocul(o)	eye	**oculo**motor – Pertaining to movements of the eye.
		intra**ocul**ar – Within the eye.

MEDICAL ROOTS / PREFIXES / SUFFIXES	MEANING	EXAMPLES
cac-	abnormal	**cac**hexia – State of ill health and malnutrition.
		cacogeusia – A bad taste not associated with something ingested.
galact(o)	milk	**galacto**phore – Milk duct.
		galactorrhea – Excessive flow of milk.
pyg(o)	buttocks	**pyg**algia – Pain of the buttocks.
sider(o)	iron	**sidero**derma – A bronze discoloration of the skin caused by a problem with iron metabolism.
		siderosis – A disease of the lungs caused by inhalation of iron.
puls(o)	drive	pro**puls**ion – Tendency to fall forward while walking.
cholangi(o)	Relating to the bile duct	**cholangio**graphy – The use of radiography to examine the bile ducts.
		cholangiectasis – Dilation of a bile duct.
dors(o)	back	**dorso**ventral – Associated with or pertaining to the back and belly.
		dorsiflexion – Bending towards the back.
electro-	amber; electrical	**electro**encephalography – Recording of changes in electric potential in various parts of the brain.
		electrolysis – Destruction by electromagnetic current.
coccyg(o)	coccyx	**coccyg**eal – Pertaining to or associated with the coccyx.
		coccygectomy – Surgical excision of the coccyx.
thi-	sulfur	**thi**ol – Sulfhydryl; containing -SH group.
ultra-	excess; beyond	**ultra**sound – Sounds greater than the limit of human hearing.
		ultrahigh – Extremely high.

MEDICAL ROOTS / PREFIXES / SUFFIXES	MEANING	EXAMPLES
palpebr(o)	eyelid	**palpebr**itis – Inflammation of the eyelid.
		palpebrate – To wink.
scaph(o)	small boat	**scaph**ocephaly – Condition of having an abnormally long and narrow skull.
		scaphoid – Boat-shaped; scaphoid bone.
vesic(o)	bladder	**vesico**vaginal – Pertaining to the bladder and vagina.
		vesicle – A small sac that is filled with fluid.
germ(o)	bud; seed; bacteria	**germ**icide – An agent that kills bacteria.
		germination – Beginning to grow.
-phyll	leaf	chloro**phyll** – Group of porphyrin derivatives that contain green magnesium; necessary for photosynthesis.
lat(o)	carry	corre**lat**e – Ability to associate one phenomena with another.
		trans**lat**e – Convert; process of codons in mRNA being converted to the sequence of amino acids constituting a polypeptide chain.
retin(o)	retina	**retin**itis – Inflammation of the retina.
		retinoschisis – Splitting of the retina.
-iasis	condition; state of; disease	cholelith**iasis** – Formation of stones in the biliary system.
		mydr**iasis** – Excessive dilation of the pupil.
varic(o)	varicose vein	**varic**oblepharon – Varicose swelling of eyelid.
		varicography – X-ray visualization of varicose veins.
amphi-	both; both sides	**amphi**arthrosis – A joint attached on both sides by fibrocartilage, allowing little motion and providing strength.
		amphibians – Vertebrates that can live both in water and on land.

MEDICAL ROOTS / PREFIXES / SUFFIXES	MEANING	EXAMPLES
syring(o)	pipe; tube; fistula	**syring**itis – Inflammation of the auditory tube.
		syringectomy – Surgical excision of a fistula.
lei(o)	smooth	**leio**dermia – Smooth skin.
		leiomyoma – A tumor that is made up of smooth muscle.
cyn(o)	dog	**cyn**ophobia – Fear of dogs.
vit(o)	life	**vito**dynamics – Pertaining to the forces of life.
		vital – To be necessary in order to live.
opt(o)	vision; eye	**opto**kinetic – Pertaining to the movement of the eye.
		optometer – A device for measuring vision.
hapl-	single	**hapl**oid – Having a single set of chromosomes.
paleo-	old	**pale**ocortex – Portion of the cerebral cortex that develops with the olfactory system and is phylogenetically older than the neocortex.
		paleopathology – Study of diseases in bodies that have been preserved since ancient times.
cholecyst(o)	gallbladder	**cholecyst**itis – Inflammation of the gallbladder.
		cholecystectomy – Surgical excision of the gallbladder.
xen(o)	foreign; strange	**xeno**genous – Caused by a foreign substance.
		xenophobia – An irrational fear of strangers.
scapul(o)	scapula	**scapulo**pexy – Surgical fixation of the scapula.
		scapulalgia – Pain of the scapular region.

MEDICAL ROOTS / PREFIXES / SUFFIXES	MEANING	EXAMPLES
ent-	inside	**ent**oblast – Endoderm.
		entoptic – Originating from within the eye.
aux(o)	increase	**aux**esis – The increase in size of an organism.
		auxilytic – To increase in destructive ability.
-opsia	vision	cyan**opsia** – A problem with the eye that causes things to appear blue.
sigmoid(o)	sigmoid	**sigmoido**tomy – Surgical incision of the sigmoid colon.
		sigmoiditis – Inflammation of the sigmoid colon.
-ad	toward; add; group; connection	caud**ad** – Toward the cauda (tail). In the human, this corresponds with the coccyx bone at the distal inferior end of the vertebral column.
		Trichomon**ad** – Parasite of genus *Trichomonas.*
infra-	below; beneath; under	**infra**structure – The basic framework; foundation.
		infrasonic – Frequency that is below the range of hearing.
-ize	a suffix which makes the word a verb	cauter**ize** – To destroy tissue by application with heat, cold, or a caustic agent.
		oxid**ize** – Cause to bond with oxygen or remove hydrogen.
rhod(o)	rose	**rhod**amine – Group of red fluorescent dyes used to label proteins.
		rhodopsin – A photosensitive purple-red chromoprotein in the retinal rods.
brachy(o)	short	**brachy**phalangia – Abnormal shortness of the phalanges.
		brachygnathia – Abnormal shortness of the lower jaw.
cyst(o)	bladder	**cyst**itis – Inflammation of the bladder.
		cystalgia – Pain in the bladder.

MEDICAL ROOTS / PREFIXES / SUFFIXES	MEANING	EXAMPLES
spasm(o)	involuntary muscle contraction; draw; pull	**spasmo**lysis – To stop muscle spasms.
il-	not; within	**il**legible – Not clear enough to be read.
		illusion – Mental impression of reality which deviates from the actual event.
enter(o)	intestine	**entero**centesis – Surgical puncture of the intestine.
		enteroparesis – Relaxation of the intestine, resulting in dilation.
anthrac(o)	coal	**anthraco**necrosis – Necrosis of tissue into a black mass.
		anthracosis – A condition due to coal dust deposition in the lungs.
cune-	wedge	**cune**iform – Wedge-shaped.
		cuneus – Wedge-shaped segment on the medial aspect of the occipital lobe of the cerebrum.
rhabd(o)	rod; striated	**rhabdo**myoma – A benign tumor made up of striated muscle.
		rhabdoviridae – A family of rod-shaped viruses.
ipsi-	self; same	**ipsi**lateral – Associated with the same side of the body.
oscill-	back and forth	**oscill**ate – To move backward and forward like a spring or pendulum.
		oscillopsia – The visual illusion that objects are swaying back and forth.
sarc(o)	flesh; connective tissue	**sarco**ma – A tumor that forms from connective tissue.
		sarcosis – The abnormal growth of flesh.
hel(o)	nail; callus	**hel**oma – A corn.
vivi-	alive	ovo**vivi**parous – Eggs are hatched within the body of the parent (e.g. snakes).

MEDICAL ROOTS / PREFIXES / SUFFIXES	MEANING	EXAMPLES
gno(s)	knowledge; know	dia**gno**sis – Knowing the cause of a problem or situation.
		pro**gno**stic – Predicting the outcome.
-lemma	husk; outer shell	sarco**lemma** – The membrane of a striated muscle cell.
dynam(o)	power	**dynam**ic – Pertaining to or associated with force.
		cardio**dynam**ics – The study of the forces associated with pumping blood in the heart.
bi-	two	**bi**lateral – Both sides.
		bicep – A muscle with two points of origin.
-phasia	speech	a**phasia** – The inability to speak.
		dys**phasia** – Difficulty speaking.
clin(o)	incline; bend; bed	**clin**ic – A place where instruction is given at the bedside.
		clinoid – Shaped like a bed.
elast(o)	elasticity	**elast**oma – Local tumorlike excess of elastic tissue fibers.
		elastometry – Measurement of elasticity.
-gram	drawing; record; letter	cardio**gram** – A drawing of the cardiac cycle used to diagnose heart disorders.
		tele**gram** – A message sent by telegraph.
sten(o)	narrow	**steno**sis – The narrowing or a duct or canal.
		stenothermic – Only thriving within a certain range of temperature (e.g. bacteria).
non-	not	**non**disjunction – Failure of chromosomes to separate correctly.
		nonspecific – Not having a known cause.

MEDICAL ROOTS / PREFIXES / SUFFIXES	MEANING	EXAMPLES
-ducent	lead; tube; duct	ab**ducent** – Serving to draw toward the medial plane or toward the axial line of a limb.
		ad**ducent** – Serving to draw away from the medial plane or from the axial line of a limb.
apo-	separation; derived from	**apo**protein – The protein portion of a molecule.
		apophysis – An outgrowth. Often used to describe bony outgrowths that do not separate from the bone (e.g. tubercle process).
gastr(o)	stomach	**gastro**pathy – A disease of the stomach.
		gastrin – A hormone that stimulates secretion of juices in the stomach.
osm(o)	smell; odor	an**osm**ia – Not having the ability to smell.
		osmophobia – The fear of odors or smells.
cymb(o)	boat	**cymb**ocephaly – Abnormal length and narrowness of the skull.
uvul(o)	uvula	**uvul**itis – Inflammation of the uvula.
		uvulectomy – Surgical excision of the uvula.
axill(o)	armpit	**axill**ary – Pertaining or related to the armpit.
		axilla – The armpit.
echin(o)	hedgehog	**echin**ocyte – A spiky cell.
tort(i)	twist; rotate	**torti**collis – A twisting of the neck to one side caused by contraction of neck muscles.
		tortellini – A pasta that is twisted into a ring-like shape and stuffed with meat or cheese.

MEDICAL ROOTS / PREFIXES / SUFFIXES	MEANING	EXAMPLES
oo(o)	egg	**oo**genesis – The development of the ova or egg.
		oocyte – An egg cell.
-phil	like; affinity for	achromato**phil** – Not having an affinity for stain; not easily stainable.
		acido**phil** – A cell or structure easily stainable with acid dyes.
crypt(o)	hide	**crypto**genic – Of an obscure origin.
		cryptomenorrhea – Menstrual systems without external bleeding.
tact(o)	touch	con**tact** – The act of touching something.
		tactile – Pertaining to touch.
noci(a)	injure	**noci**ceptor – Receptor for pain.
occip(o)	back of the head	**occip**ut – The back of the head.
arteri(o)	artery	**arterio**sclerosis – Hardening of the arteries.
		arteritis – Inflammation of one or more arteries.
lip(o)	fat	**lipo**lysis – The breakdown of fat.
		lipoid – To resemble fat.
tub(o)	pipe	**tubo**plasty – Plastic repair of a tube (e.g. uterine or auditory).
icter(o)	jaundice	**ictero**genic – Causing jaundice.
		icterohepatitis – Inflammation or the liver marked by jaundice.
phe(o)	dusky	**pheo**chrome – Stained darkly with chromium salts.
carp(o)	wrist	**carp**us – The wrist.
		carpectomy – Excision of a wrist bone.

MEDICAL ROOTS / PREFIXES / SUFFIXES	MEANING	EXAMPLES
splen(o)	spleen	**spleno**megaly – Enlargement of the spleen.
		splenopexy – Surgical fixation of the spleen.
ech(o)	have; hold	syn**ech**ia – An adhesion, as of the iris to the cornea or lens.
blast(o)	bud; early stages of growth	**blasto**cyte – A primary germ cell.
		blastotomy – Separation of cells during the early stages of human development.
schiz(o)	split; divide	**schizo**phrenia – A mental disorder characterized by split personalities.
		schizonychia – Splitting of the nails.
prote(o)	protein	**prote**inase – An enzyme that breaks down a protein.
		proteinemia – An excess of protein in the blood.
trep(o)	turn	**trep**opnea – Difficult breathing that is relieved when the patient is lying on the side.
furc(o)	fork	**furc**ula – A forked bone, the wishbone or furculum.
		furcation – To branch like a fork.
taenia-	pertaining to tapeworms	**taenia**cide – Destroys tapeworms.
		taeniafuge – Expels tapeworms.
-plasia	formation; growth	hyper**plasia** – Excessive growth.
		achondro**plasia** – Improper growth of cartilage.
-scope	to examine	endo**scope** – An instrument for viewing an inner part of the body.
		stetho**scope** – A instrument used for listening to the sounds of the chest.

MEDICAL ROOTS / PREFIXES / SUFFIXES	MEANING	EXAMPLES
glutin(o)	glue	ag**glutin**ant – Causes adhesive union; substance that holds parts together during healing.
		glutinous – Adhesive.
lev(o)	left	**lev**orotatory – Turning the plane of polarization of polarized light to the left.
ampulla	dilation of a tubular structure	**ampulla** of vater – The dilation of the pancreatic and common bile ducts as they merge before entering the duodenum.
		ampulla membranaceae – Dilation at the end of each semicircular duct.
oc-	against	**oc**clusion – A blockage; trapping of liquid or gas within cavities; Relation of the teeth when in contact; momentary closure of the vocal tract.
		occult – Obscure; hidden.
hymen(o)	membrane	**hymen** – A membrane that covers part of the entrance to the vagina.
		hymenology – The study of the membranes of the body.
sphygm(o)	pulse	**sphygmo**manometer – An instrument that measures arterial blood pressure.
		sphygmoid – Resembling the pulse.
fec(o)	feces	**fec**ulent – Pertaining to or associated with feces.
		fecalith – A hard mass of feces.
e-	out from	**e**motion – A strong feeling state directed toward a specific object.
		emission – Discharge.
sinistr(o)	left	**sinistro**cular – Being dominant in the left eye.
		sinistropedal – Using the left foot over the right foot.

MEDICAL ROOTS / PREFIXES / SUFFIXES	MEANING	EXAMPLES
umbilic(o)	navel	**umbilic**al – Pertaining to the navel.
		umbilication – Resembling the navel.
bacteri(o)	bacteria	**bacteri**cidal – Something that kills bacteria.
		bacteremia – Bacteria in the blood.
fract(o)	break	**fract**al – Curve or geometric figure, each part of which has the same statistical character as the whole.
		fracture – Breaking of a part (e.g. bone).
sin(o)	sinus; hollow tube	**sino**bronchitis – Inflammation of the paranasal sinus along with bronchial inflammation.
		sinoatrial – Relating to the sinoatrial node of the heart.
necr(o)	death; corpse	**necro**sis – The death of tissue.
		necrophobia – Fear of death or dead bodies.
sterc(o)	feces	**sterco**roma – A mass of fecal matter that is tumor-like.
		stercolith – A hard mass of fecal matter.
dolich-	long	**dolich**ocephalic – Long headed.
cine(o)	movement	**cine**matography – The making of a motion picture or film.
		cineradiography – Making a motion picture of successive x-rays.
ten(o)	tendon	**teno**plasty – Surgical repair of a tendon.
		tenodesis – Surgical fixation of a tendon to a bone.
vers(o)	turn	con**vers**ion – Change; transformation.

MEDICAL ROOTS / PREFIXES / SUFFIXES	MEANING	EXAMPLES
sperm(at)	semen	**spermat**ogenesis – The production of sperm.
		spermicide – An agent that kills sperm.
hidr(o)	sweat	**hidro**tic – Sweating an abnormal amount.
		dys**hidro**sis – A disorder of the sweat glands.
lax(a)	loosen; widen	**laxa**tive – Something that widens the intestinal tract or loosens stool.
		re**lax** – To make less tense or loosen the muscles.
pend(o)	hang	ap**pend**age – A suboordinate outgrowth of a structure.
		ap**pend**ix – A supplementary, accessory, or dependent part of a main structure.
aneurysm(o)	a dilation of the wall of an artery, vein, or the heart	**aneurysm**ectomy – Surgical excision of the aneurysm.
		aneurysmoplasty – Surgical repair of the aneurysm.
retro-	backward; behind	**retro**grade – To go backwards.
		retroflex – To bend backwards.
hod(o)	path	**hod**oneuromere – Segment of the embryonic trunk.
bili-	bile	**bili**rubin – A bile pigment.
		biliary atresia – Lack or obliteration of the bile duct.
rhin(o)	nose	**rhino**plasty – Plastic surgery of the nose.
		rhinorrhea – Discharge of fluid through the nose.
contra-	opposite; against	**contra**rian – An individual who opposes the position taken by the majority.
		contralateral – Affecting the opposite side.
palin-	recurring	**palin**dromia – Happening again.
		palinopsia – Preservation of a visual sensation after the stimulus is gone.

MEDICAL ROOTS / PREFIXES / SUFFIXES	MEANING	EXAMPLES
-ase	a suffix denoting an enzyme	protein**ase** – An enzyme that breaks down a protein.
		lip**ase** – An enzyme that breaks down a fat.
jejun(o)	empty; jejunum	gastro**jejuno**stomy – Surgery to make a new passage between the stomach and jejunum.
		jejunotomy – Surgical incision of the jejunum.
poster(o)	back; behind	**poster**ior – Situated at the back; opposite of anterior.
		posteroanterior – Extending from the back to the front.
disc(o)	disk	**disc**ogenic – Caused by derangement of an intervertebral disk.
		discoplacenta – Discoid placenta.
-coccus	berry	staphylo**coccus** – A round shaped gram-positive bacteria that is usually found in clusters like grapes.
		strepto**coccus** – A round shaped bacteria that usually occurs in pairs or strains.
brom(o)	stench; foul odor	**brom**hidrosis – Sweat that has a foul odor.
		bromomenorrhea – Menstruation that has an offensive odor.
-phobia	fear; dread	necro**phobia** – Fear of death or dead bodies.
		gyne**phobia** – Fear of women.
ectr(o)	miscarriage; congenital absence	**ectro**dactyly – Absence of a finger or toe.
		ectrogeny – The absence or defect of a part.
-plasm	formation; growth substance	neo**plasm** – A new and abnormal growth.
		nucleo**plasm** – The protoplasm found in the nucleus of a cell.

MEDICAL ROOTS / PREFIXES / SUFFIXES	MEANING	EXAMPLES
-ar	relating or pertaining to	cardiovascul**ar** – Related to the heart and vasculature.
		follicul**ar** – Related to one or more follicles.
-itis	inflammation	cyst**itis** – Inflammation of the bladder.
		bronch**itis** – Inflammation of one or more bronchi.
ger(o)	old age	**ger**iatrics – Medicine that deals with the elderly.
		gerodontics – Dentistry that deals with the elderly.
vuls(o)	twitch	con**vuls**ion – Involuntary contractions of voluntary muscle; seizure.
thromb(o)	clot	**thrombo**cytopenia – An abnormally low number of platelets in the blood.
		thrombogenesis – Clot formation.
pector(o)	chest	ex**pector**ation – To cough up mucous and phlegm from the chest.
		pectoral – Pertaining to the chest or breast.
chron(o)	time	ana**chron**ism – Not in the correct historical time; out of chronological order.
		chronic – Constant; existing for a long time.
hal(o)	breath	ex**hal**e – To breathe out.
		halitosis – Bad breath.
somat(o)	body	**somat**ic – Pertaining to the body.
		psycho**somat**ic – Pertaining to or involving both the mind and the body.
bol(o)	throw; ball	em**bol**ism – Blocking of an artery by a clot or object brought via blood flow.
		bolus – A rounded mass of food or pharmaceutical preparation made ready to swallow.

MEDICAL ROOTS / PREFIXES / SUFFIXES	MEANING	EXAMPLES
muc(o)	mucus	**muc**inosis – Having an elevated amount of mucins in the skin.
		mucopurulent – Having both mucus and pus.
didym(o)	twin; testis	**didymo**us – Existing in pairs or twins.
		epi**didym**is – The structure where sperm are stored.
lyo-	loose; dissolve	**lyo**philic – Stable in solution.
		lyophobic – Unstable in solution.
scrot(o)	scrotum	**scroto**cele – A hernia of the scrotum.
		scrotectomy – Surgical excision of the scrotum.
arch(e)	first; origin	patri**arch** – A man considered to be a father or founder.
		men**arche** – The onset of menstruation.
phrax(i)	wall; fence	salpingem**phrax**is – Obstruction of an auditory tube.
lob(o)	lobe	**lob**ectomy – Surgical excision of a lobe.
		lobation – Forming of lobes.
ad-	to, when not preceding the consonants *c,f,g,p,s*, or *t*	**ad**duct – Movement toward the midline of a structure. To adduct the arm is to bring it down the side of the body. To adduct the fingers is to bring them together so they are closer to the midline of the upper extremity.
		adneural – Toward a nerve (as electric current passes from muscle to nerve).
scot(o)	darkness	**scoto**phobia – An abnormal fear of the dark.
		scotopia – The ability to see in dim light.

MEDICAL ROOTS / PREFIXES / SUFFIXES	MEANING	EXAMPLES
cor(o)	pupil; with; together	**cor**nea – The transparent part of the eye.
		corectasis – Dilation of the pupil.
		correlate – Ability to associate one phenomena with another.
drom(o)	course	**dromo**graph – A instrument for recording the rate at which blood flows through the body.
		syn**drome** – A set of symptoms that together characterize a disease; they "run their course together."
bi(o)	life	aero**bi**c – Living in the presence of molecular oxygen.
		biogenesis – The origin of life.
encephal(o)	brain	**encephalo**pathy – Any pathological condition affecting the brain.
		encephalitis – Inflammation of the brain.
-poietic	formation of	sarco**poietic** – The formation of muscle.
		myelo**poietic** – The formation of bone marrow.
cancr(o)	cancer	**cancr**oid – Resembling cancer.
nucle(o)	nucleus	**nucleo**plasm – The protoplasm found in the nucleus of a cell.
		nucleoprotein – Proteins found in the nucleus of a cell.
corp(o)	body	**corp**se – A dead body.
sphen(o)	wedge; sphenoid bone	**spheno**id – Wedge-shaped.
		sphenoiditis – Inflammation of the sphenoid sinus.
chir(o)	hand; also spelled cheir-	**chiro**plasty – Plastic surgery on the hand.
		chiromegaly – Enlargement of the hands.

MEDICAL ROOTS / PREFIXES / SUFFIXES	MEANING	EXAMPLES
rot(o)	wheel	**rot**ablation – Atherectomy technique in which a rotating burr is placed through a catheter into an artery.
		rotate – To turn around an axis.
stern(o)	sternum; breastbone	**stern**algia – Pain in the sternum.
		sternoschisis – A splitting of the sternum.
pan-	all	**pan**demic – Universal; a disease found throughout.
		pancytopenia – A lack of all blood cells.
norm(o)	usual; pattern	**normo**tensive – Having normal blood pressure.
		normocyte – An erythrocyte that is normal according to size, shape, and color.
creat(o)	meat	**creat**ine – Amino acid which occurs mostly in muscle tissue and is important in storing high-energy phosphate.
splanchn(o)	viscera	**splanchno**logy – The study of the viscera of the body.
		splanchnicectomy – Surgical excision of one or more splanchnic nerves.
for(o)	bore	imper**for**ate – Abnormally closed.
		foramen – Naturally occuring opening or passage (e.g. into bone).
articul(o)	joint	**articul**ation – A joint between two bones.
		articulate – Divided by joints.
syn-	with; together	**syn**desis – To bind together.
		syndrome – A set of symptoms that together characterize a disease. They "run their course together."

MEDICAL ROOTS / PREFIXES / SUFFIXES	MEANING	EXAMPLES
phys(o)	wind; inflate	**phys**ometra – Gas in the uterine cavity.
		em**phys**ema – Irregular accumulation of air in tissues or organs.
mast(o)	breast	hyper**mast**ia – Enlargement of the breasts.
		mastectomy – Surgical removal of the breast.
seb(o)	sebaceous; fat; grease	**sebo**rrhea – An abnormal discharge from the sebaceous glands.
		sebum – The oil that is secreted through the sebaceous glands.
thigm(o)	touch	**thigm**otaxis – Causing movement by response to contact or touch.
cox-	hip	**cox**algia – Pain in the hip.
		coxa – The hip.
-plasty	mold; shape; surgical repair	mento**plasty** – Plastic surgery on the chin.
		chiro**plasty** – Plastic surgery on the hand.
in(o)	fiber	**in**otropic – Affecting the force of muscular contractions.
nephr(o)	kidney	**nephro**lithotripsy – Removal of kidney stones.
		nephrology – The study of the kidneys.
rhiz(o)	root	**rhizo**tomy – Cutting of the spinal nerve roots.
		rhizoid – To resemble a root.
posit(o)	put; place	de**posit** – Sediment; inorganic matter collecting in an organ or a body.
en-	in; on	**en**clave – An area or group that is isolated within a larger one.
		endural – Within the ear.
jugul(o)	neck	**jugul**ar – Of or pertaining to the neck or throat.

MEDICAL ROOTS / PREFIXES / SUFFIXES	MEANING	EXAMPLES
stol(o)	send	dia**stol**e – Dialation of the heart's ventricles.
		pi**stol** – The smallest firearm intended to be fired with one hand.
pro-	before; forward	**pro**hibit – To stop before something happens.
		progression – To move forward.
fibr(o)	fiber	**fibro**ma – A tumor composed of mainly fibrous tissue.
		fibrochondritis – Inflammation of fibrocartilage.
phen(o)	show	**pheno**type – Observable characteristics of an individual.
ossi-	bone	**ossi**ferous – Producing bone.
		ossicle – A small bone.
neo-	new; young	**neo**natal – Pertaining to a newborn child.
		neoplasm – A new and abnormal growth.
endo-	inside	**endo**derm – The innermost germ layer of the embryo.
		endometrium – The lining within the uterus.
clus-	shut	in**clus**ion – The act of closing; being closed.
		oc**clus**ion – Obstruction; trapped liquids or gases; relation of teeth on each jaw when in contact; closure of some area of the vocal tract.
amyl(o)	starch	**amylo**id – A substance resembling starch that is deposited in several disease states.
		amylose – A carbohydrate (except glucose or saccharose).
de-	down; lack of	**de**compression – To remove pressure.
		degeneration – Going to higher to lower; declining.

MEDICAL ROOTS / PREFIXES / SUFFIXES	MEANING	EXAMPLES
eosin(o)	red; rosy	**eosino**penia – A low number of eosinophils in the blood.
		eosinophil – A white blood cell that stains with red dye.
steth(o)	chest	**stetho**scope – A instrument used for listening to the sounds of the chest.
		stethospasm – Spasm of the chest muscles.
log(o)	speak; speech	**log**apathy – A speech disorder.
		logoplegia – Paralysis of speech organs.
fug(i)	flee	**fug**ue – State of altered consciousness in which the individual wanders aimlessly, not guided by his normal personality and which is not remembered afterwards.
		centri**fug**ation – Process of separating heavy particles from lighter particles using centrifugal force.
cauter(o)	burn	**cauter**y – An instrument that destroys tissue by burning.
		cauterize – To burn with a cautery.
phren(o)	mind; diaphragm	**phreno**plegia – Paralysis of the diaphragm.
		schizo**phren**ia – A mental disorder characterized by split personalities.
tuber(o)	swelling; node	**tuber**cle – Nodule or small projection.
ungu(o)	nail	sub**ungu**al – Beneath the nail.
		ungual – Pertaining to the nails.
burs(o)	fluid-filled sac	**burs**a – A fluid-filled sac.
		bursitis – Inflammation of a bursa.
-cleisis	enclose	colpo**cleisis** – Surgical closure of the vaginal cavity.

MEDICAL ROOTS / PREFIXES / SUFFIXES	MEANING	EXAMPLES
tox(o)	poison	**tox**emia – Poisoned blood caused by bacteria.
		toxicity – The state of being poisonous.
mega-	large; great	**mega**logastria – An abnormally large stomach.
		megacystis – An enlarged bladder.
phthi(a)	decay	**phthi**sis – A wasting away of the body.
-ia	state; condition; quality of	eupeps**ia** – Good or normal digestion.
		anem**ia** – Lack of red blood cells.
anthrop(o)	man	**anthropo**logy – The study of man.
		anthropometer – An instrument that measures body dimensions.
oneir(o)	dream	**oneir**ism – Waking dream state.
stomat(o)	mouth	**stomato**menia – Bleeding of the mouth during menstruation.
		stomatomalacia – A softening of the mouth.
gluc(o)	pertaining to or associated with glucose	**gluco**neogenesis – The production of glucose.
		glucophore – An amino derivative of glucose.
-sthenia	strength	mya**sthenia** – A lack of muscular strength.
		eu**sthenia** – Having normal strength.
phlog(o)	burn	**phlog**ogenic – Causing inflammation.
act-	do; drive	re**act**ion – Chemical process in which one or more substances are changed into different substances.
		active transport – Movement of ions or molecules across a cell membrane into a region of higher concentration at the cost of energy.

MEDICAL ROOTS / PREFIXES / SUFFIXES	MEANING	EXAMPLES
-nychia	nail	pachyo**nychia** – Thickening of the nails.
		ano**nychia** – Not having fingernails.
thym(o)	thymus gland	**thym**ectomy – Surgical excision of the thymus.
		thymocyte – A white blood cell that arises from the thymus.
arteriol(o)	arteriole; a small artery	**arteriolo**necrosis – Degeneration of arterioles.
		arteriolosclerosis – Hardening of arterioles.
granul(o)	granular; grainy	**granulo**cytopenia – A decrease in granular leukocytes.
		granuloma – A tumor composed of granular tissue.
cleid(o)	clavicle	**cleid**ocranial – Pertaining to the clavicle and the head.
lumb(o)	loin; lower back	**lumbo**sacral – Associated with or pertaining to the loins and sacrum.
		lumbar – Associated with or pertaining to the lower back.
pauci-	few	**pauci**synaptic – Involving only a few synapses in series.
xer(o)	dry	**xero**derma – To have dry skin.
		xeroma – A dryness of the conjunctiva of the eye.
brevi-	short	**brevi**collis – Shortness of the neck.
		brevirostrate – A short beak.
sudo-	pertaining to sweat	**sudo**motor – To stimulate the sweat glands.
jact(i)	throw	**jact**itation – Restless back and forth or side to side movement during acute illness.
somn(o)	sleep	**somn**ambulism – Sleepwalking.
		in**somni**ac – A person who has difficulty sleeping.

MEDICAL ROOTS / PREFIXES / SUFFIXES	MEANING	EXAMPLES
nyct(o)	night	**nyct**alopia – Night blindness.
		nyctophobia – Fear of darkness.
press(o)	press; force	**press**or – Tending to increase blood pressure.
		pressure – Force per unit area.
-lepsy	seizure; attack; uncontrolled	narco**lepsy** – A disorder that causes uncontrolled episodes of deep sleep.
		epi**lepsy** – A disorder of the nervous system that causes brain malfunction and often results in seizures.
anis(o)	unequal; not similar	**aniso**coria – Having pupils that are different in size.
		anisopiesis – Having varying blood pressure in different parts of the body.
tors(o)	twist; rotate	**tors**ion – Twisting or rotating around an axis.
		torso – Trunk.
multi-	many; much	**multi**para – A woman who has had two or more pregnancies.
		multinodular – Having many nodules.
extra-	outside of; beyond	**extra**terrestrial – Located outside of the earth.
		extrarenal – Located outside of the kidney.
vir(i)	male; masculine	**viri**le – Masculine.
		virilism – The development of male characteristics.
cis-	same side	**cis**platin – A platinum complex used to create interstrand DNA crosslinks.
lute(o)	yellow	**lute**in – A yellow pigment.
		luteoma – A yellow tumor found in the ovary.

MEDICAL ROOTS / PREFIXES / SUFFIXES	MEANING	EXAMPLES
zo-	animal	**zo**ology – The study of animals.
		zoodermic – Done using the skin of an animal.
phag(o)	eat	**phago**cyte – A cell that ingests foreign particles.
		poly**phago**us – Eating many types of food.
cata-	negative; against; down	**cata**bolism – The breaking down of complex substances into more simple substances.
		catagen – A portion of the hair cycle in which growth stops.
-opsy	to view	aut**opsy** – To inspect a body after death to determine the cause.
		bi**opsy** – To examine a piece of tissue from the body for diagnosis.
xiph(o)	sword; xiphoid process	**xipho**iditis – Inflammation of the xiphoid process.
		xiphocostal – Pertaining to the xiphoid process and the ribs.
ambul(o)	walk	**ambul**atory – The ability to walk; not bedridden.
		ambulance – A "walking hospital."
hist(o)	tissue	**histo**kinesis – Movement of tissues in the body.
		histology – The study of tissues in the body.
dicty(o)	nest	**dicty**otene – Stage in which the primary oocyte spends from late fetal life until discharged from ovary.
platy-	broad; flat	**platy**podia – Flat-footed.
		platyhelminthes – Flatworms.
follicul(o)	follicle	**follicul**ar – Related to one or more follicles.
		folliculitis – Inflammation of a follicle.

MEDICAL ROOTS / PREFIXES / SUFFIXES	MEANING	EXAMPLES
copr(o)	feces	**copro**phobia – Fear of feces.
		coprostasis – Fecal impactation in the intestine.
hapt(o)	touch	**hapt**ics – Study of the sense of touch.
-ectomy	to take out	append**ectomy** – Surgical excision of the vermiform appendix.
		hyster**ectomy** – Surgical excision of the uterus.
spin(o)	spine	**spino**cerebellar – Pertaining to the spine and the cerebellum.
		spinal – Pertaining to or associated with the spine.
antr(o)	cavity	**antr**itis – Inflammation of an antrum, often describing the maxillary sinus (antrum).
		antrotymanic – Relating to the tympanic antrum and tympanum (middle ear cavity).
rhytid-	wrinkle	**rhytid** – A wrinkle in the skin.
		rhytidectomy – Surgical excision of skin to remove wrinkles.
gingiv(o)	gum	**gingiv**itis – Inflammation of the gums.
		gingiva – The gum.
occipit(o)	pertaining to the occipital region of the skull	**occipito**parietal – Pertaining to the occipital and parietal bones or lobes of the skull.
cirs(o)	varix (varicose vessels)	**cirs**oid – Resembling a varix (a large twisting blood or lymphatic vessel).
metr(o)	uterus; womb	**metro**plasty – Plastic surgery on the uterus.
		metrorrhea – An abnormal discharge from the uterus.
bar(o)	weight	**baro**trauma – Injury caused by a change in pressure.
		barometer – An instrument for determining weight or pressure of the atmosphere.

MEDICAL ROOTS / PREFIXES / SUFFIXES	MEANING	EXAMPLES
poikil(o)	spotted; irregular; varied	**poikilo**derma – Any skin disorder characterized by patchy discolorations.
		poikilocytosis – A condition which is characterized by varied cell shapes.
rubr(o)	red	**rubr**ospinal – Pertaining to the red nucleus and the spinal cord.
febr(o)	fever	a**febr**ile – Without fever.
		febricity – Having a fever.
juxta-	near; beside	**juxta**position – Side by side.
iatr(o)	physician	pedi**atr**ician – A physician who treats children.
		iatrogenic – Caused by the medical treatment of a physician.
aque(o)	water	**aque**duct – A canal or channel.
		aqueous – Watery.
-ject	throw	inter**ject** – To speak abruptly; an interruption.
neur(o)	nerve	**neur**ectopia – Abnormal placement of a nerve.
		neuralgia – Sharp pain along the course of a nerve.
bis-	twice	**bis**albuminemia – A condition in which two types of albumin are present in an individual.
		bisiliac – Associated with the two iliac bones.
funct(o)	perform	de**funct** – Dead; no longer existing or able to function.
tel(o)	end	**telo**phase – The final stage of mitosis.
		telomere – The end of a eukaryotic chromosome.
gon(o)	offspring; genitalia; knee	**gon**ad – Gamete producing gland (e.g. ovary or testis).
		gonarthritis – Inflammation of the knee.

MEDICAL ROOTS / PREFIXES / SUFFIXES	MEANING	EXAMPLES
pet(o)	move toward	centri**pet**al – Toward a center.
insul(o)	island	**insul**in – A hormone that is produced by the islets of Langerhans.
		insulate – To surround or make an island of.
kine(o)	movement	hyper**kine**sia – Excessive movement.
		kinesitherapy – The treatment of disease through massage and exercise.
chyl(i)	juice	**chyl**e – The milky fluid taken up by the lacteals from food in the instestine.
		chyliform – Resembling chyle.
lingu(o)	tongue	bi**lingu**al – Speaking two languages.
		sub**lingu**al – Beneath the tongue.
strept(o)	twist	**strepto**coccus – A round shaped bacteria that usually occurs in pairs or strains.
andr(o)	male	**andro**gen – A substance that induces male characteristics (e.g. testosterone).
		androblastoma – A benign tumor of the testicles.
tract(o)	draw; drag	**tract**ion – Act of drawing or pulling.
cyt(o)	cell	**cyto**kinesis – Final stage of cell division when the cytoplasm splits.
		cytology – The study of cells.
phos-	light	**phos**e – Any visual stimulus such as light or color.
dendr(o)	tree; branching	**dendro**logy – The study of trees.
		dendrite – One of the branches of a nerve cell that receives impulses.
ul(o)	scar; gum	**ul**erythema – Erythematous skin disease with scarring and atrophy.
		ulotomy – Incision of scar tissue; incision of the gums.

MEDICAL ROOTS / PREFIXES / SUFFIXES	MEANING	EXAMPLES
ot(o)	ear	par**ot**id – The salivary gland of the ear.
		otorrhea – Discharge from the ear.
jug(u)	yoke; neck	con**jug**ate – Paired; working together.
		jugular – Of or pertaining to the neck or throat.
onych(o)	nail	**onych**omycosis – A fungal infection of the nails.
-phylaxis	protection	chemopro**phylaxis** – Protection against disease by means of chemicals agents.
lept(o)	thin; slender; delicate	**lepto**cephalus – Having an abnormally narrow skull.
		leptotene – A stage of cell division which occurs during prophase of meiosis I in which the chromosomes are threadlike.
chol(e)	bile	**chol**agogue – A substance that causes bladder contraction in order to promote bile flow.
		cholelithiasis – Formation of stones in the biliary system.
uni-	one	**uni**lateral – Having one side.
		unicellular – Made up of a single cell.
phyc(o)	seaweed	**Phyc**omycetes – Group of fungi which are common water, leaf, and bread molds.
		phycology – Study of seaweeds and other algae.
myring(o)	membrane; eardrum	**myringo**plasty – Surgical repair of the eardrum.
		myringectomy – Surgical excision of the eardrum.
butyr(o)	butter	**butyr**oid – Resembling butter.
vir(o)	virus; poison	**vir**uria – Having viruses in the urine.
		virolactia – Secretion of viruses in milk.

MEDICAL ROOTS / PREFIXES / SUFFIXES	MEANING	EXAMPLES
digit-	finger; toe	**digit**al – Performed with the fingers.
		inter**digit**ate – To weave or interlock like fingers do when holding hands.
pub(o)	adult	**pub**erty – The age when the secondary sexual characters develop allowing for the ability to sexually reproduce.
		ischio**pub**ic – Pertaining to the ischium and pubes.
thyr(o)	thyroid gland	**thyro**megaly – An enlarged thyroid gland.
		thyrotropin – Thyroid stimulating hormone.
men(o)	menstruation	hypo**meno**rrhea – A decreased menstrual flow.
		menarche – The onset of menstruation.
pelv(i)	pelvis	**pelvi**otomy – Surgical incision of the pelvic bone.
		pelvimetry – Measurement of the pelvis.
son(o)	sound	**son**ication – The disruption of bacteria by exposure to sound waves that are high in frequency.
		sonogram – The image of a fetus produced by reflecting sound waves.
gyr(o)	ring; circle	**gyr**ospasm – Spasm in which the head rotates around the neck.
		gyrate – Revolve around a fixed point.
loc-	place	**loc**ator – Device used for determining the site of foreign objects in the body.
		trans**loc**ation – Movement of a substance from one site to another.
bronch(o)	windpipe; bronchus	**bronch**itis – Inflammation of one or more bronchi.
		bronchial – Pertaining to or associated with one or more bronchi.

MEDICAL ROOTS / PREFIXES / SUFFIXES	MEANING	EXAMPLES
-plegia	paralysis	logo**plegia** – Paralysis of speech organs.
		irido**plegia** – Paralysis of the sphincter of the iris.
-on	goes; moves	electr**on** – Negatively charged particle.
		positr**on** – Positively charged particle.
dia-	apart; through; between; complete	**dia**meter – The distance through the center of a circle.
		diarrhea – The flowing through of watery feces.
pher(o)	support; outer edge; outside	peri**pher**y – An outward surface or structure; an outer edge.
		pheromone – Substance secreted to the outside of the body which elicits a certain behavior in other individuals of the same species.
viscer(o)	internal organ	**viscero**megaly – Enlargement of an internal organ.
		visceralgia – Pain of a viscera.
pancreat(o)	pancreas	**pancreat**ectomy – Surgical excision of the pancreas.
		pancreatotropic – Having an affinity for the pancreas.
bulb(o)	bulb	**bulb**ospiral – In reference to certain cardiac muscle pertaining to the root of the aorta and having a spiral course.
coron(o)	associated with or pertaining to the coronary arteries; crown-shaped	**coron**ary – Encircling like a crown; associated with the heart.
		coronoid – Crown-shaped.
-phagia	eating	oligo**phagia** – Eating only a few types of food.
		hyper**phagia** – Constantly hungry.
nutri(o)	nourish	mal**nutri**tion – Not having good nutrition.
		nutrient – A nourishing substance.

MEDICAL ROOTS / PREFIXES / SUFFIXES	MEANING	EXAMPLES
spor(o)	seed	**spor**ocyst – Cyst or sac containing reproductive cells.
		zoo**spor**e – Motile, flagellated spore produced by algae, fungi, or protozoa.
esthe(s)	feeling; sensation	an**esthesia** – The loss of sensation.
		hyp**esthesia** – A decrease in sensation.
herpet(o)	crawl; snake	**herpet**ology – Study of snakes.
-grade	movement; walk; go	retro**grade** – To go backwards.
		up**grade** – To go upwards.
-ic	associated with; pertaining to	geriatr**ics** – Medicine that deals with the elderly.
lecith(o)	yolk	iso**lecith**al – Yolk evenly distributed throughout the cytoplasm as in mammalian eggs.
		lecithal – Having yolk.
ather(o)	relating or pertaining to cholesterol and fatty plaques found within the inner surface of arteries	**athero**sclerosis – A type of arteriosclerosis involving atheroma formation in arteries.
		atheroma – An intraluminal arterial plaque composed of cholesterol and lipid material.
polio-	gray	**polio**clastic – Destruction of the gray matter of the nervous system.
		polioencephalitis – A disease of the gray matter in the brain.
typ(o)	type	**typ**ology – Study of types; science of classifying according to type.
-opia	vision	dipl**opia** – Having double vision.

MEDICAL ROOTS / PREFIXES / SUFFIXES	MEANING	EXAMPLES
pros(o)	front	**pros**odemic – Direct transmission of a disease from one person to another.
		prosoplasia – Abnormal differentiation of tissue; Development into a higher level of organization or function.
di-	two; double	**di**ataxia – Loss of coordination of muscles on both sides of the body.
		diarthric – Pertaining to or affecting two different joints.
sacr(o)	sacrum	**sacr**algia – Pain in the sacrum.
		sacrospinal – Pertaining to the sacrum and spinal column.
lymphaden(o)	lymph nodes	**lymphadeno**cele – Cyst on the lymph node.
		lymphadenitis – Inflammation of a lymph node.
chore(o)	dance	**chore**a – A condition characterized by rapid, jerky, involuntary movements.
		choreography – A sequence of movements, as in dance.
prostat(o)	prostate gland	**prostato**megaly – Enlargement of the prostate gland.
		prostatodynia – Pain of the prostate gland.
aur(o)	ear	**aur**icle – The appendage of the ear.
		auriculotemporal – Pertaining or related to the region of the ear and temple.
phalang(o)	phalanges; fingers; toes	**phalang**ectomy – Surgical excision of a finger or toe.
		inter**phalang**eal – Between the fingers or toes.
zyg(o)	union; yoke	**zygo**te – The union of two gametes or a fertilized egg.
		zygosis – Conjugation.
leuk(o)	white	**leuko**cyte – White blood cell.
		leukoplakia – White patches on the mucous membrane.

MEDICAL ROOTS / PREFIXES / SUFFIXES	MEANING	EXAMPLES
spir(o)	coil; breathing	re**spir**ation – The act of breathing.
		spirochete – A microorganism that is coil-shaped.
ped(i)	child	**pedi**atrician – A physician who treats children.
atre-	closed	biliary **atre**sia – Lack or obliteration of the bile duct.
physi(o)	nature	**physio**logy – The study of the functions of living organisms.
		physiography – The study of the earth's natural features.
-ostomy	mouth; artificial or surgical opening	col**ostomy** – A surgical operation to create an artificial anus.
		gastrojejun**ostomy** – Surgery to make a new passage between the stomach and jejunum.
acet(o)	vinegar	**acet**ic – Pertaining to vinegar; sour
-globin	protein	hemo**globin** – A protein found in red blood cells.
		myo**globin** – A protein found in the muscle.
ur(o)	urine	lith**ur**esis – Small stones in the urine.
		semin**ur**ia – The presence of semen in the urine.
maxill(o)	upper jaw	**maxillo**mandibular – Associated with or pertaining to the upper and lower jaws.
		sub**maxill**ary – Beneath the jaw.
tele-	distance	**tele**kinesis – The movement of an object without contact.
		teletherapy – Treatment in which the agent does not contact the body.
cav-	hollow	**cav**ernous – Pertaining to or associated with a hollow space.
		cavity – A hollow place inside the body.

MEDICAL ROOTS / PREFIXES / SUFFIXES	MEANING	EXAMPLES
stear(o)	fat	**stear**ic acid – Saturated fatty acid found in most fats or oils.
koil(o)	hollow	**koilo**cyte – A hollow cell.
		koilonychia – A condition in which the fingernails are concave and have raised edges.
inter-	among; between	**inter**nal – Found on the inside.
		interaction – Action between individuals or substances.
fund(i)	pour	in**fundi**bulum – Funnel shaped structure.
		fundiform – Shaped like a loop or sling.
ureter(o)	ureter	**ureter**ectasis – Dilation of the ureter.
		ureterolith – A calculus in the ureter.
ambo-	both	**ambo**n – The cartilaginous ring around a bone socket containing the head of a long bone.
		amboceptor – The double receptor of hemolysin.
proct(o)	anus	**procto**plegia – Paralysis of the rectum.
		proctotomy – Surgical incision of the rectum.
styl(o)	stake; pillar; poke	**stylo**id – Resembling a pillar; relating to the styloid process.
		stylohyoid – Pertaining to the styloid process and hyoid bone.
hex(o)	have; be	cac**hex**ia – State of ill health and malnutrition.
gynec(o)	woman	**gyneco**logy – A branch of medicine dealing with women.
		gynephobia – Fear of women.

MEDICAL ROOTS / PREFIXES / SUFFIXES	MEANING	EXAMPLES
kal(i)	potassium	**kali**uresis – Potassium in the urine.
		hyper**kal**emia – An elevated amount of potassium in the blood.
calc(o)	stone-like; heel; calcium	**calc**aneus – The heel bone.
		calcification – Hardening of tissue due to calcium deposition.
deuter-	second	**deuter**anomaly – Most common color vision deficiency in which the second green-sensitive cones have decreased sensitivity.
		deuteropathy – Disease that is secondary to another disease.
sopor(o)	deep sleep	**sopor**ific – To induce sleep.
		sopor – An unnaturally deep sleep.
lien(o)	spleen	gastro**lien**al – Pertaining to the stomach and the spleen.
		lienomalacia – Softening of the spleen.
phyl(o)	group; same kind	**phyl**ogeny – Developmental history of organisms.
hyper-	beyond; above	**hyper**emesis – Excessive vomiting.
		hyperglycemia – Elevated blood sugar level.
cortic(o)	bark; outer layer; cortex	**cortico**trophin – A hormone that stimulates the adrenal cortex.
		corticolous – Living on bark.
angina	"squeezing" pain, often associated with lack of oxygen to the heart	**angina** pectoris – Pain associated with lack of oxygen to the heart.
		intestinal **angina** – Spasmodic pain associated with lack of oxygen to the abdominal viscera.
poly-	many; much	**poly**chromatic – Having many colors.
		polyphagous – Eating many types of food.

MEDICAL ROOTS / PREFIXES / SUFFIXES	MEANING	EXAMPLES
opisth(o)	backward; behind	**opistho**tonos – A spasm that causes the body to bend backwards.
		opisthognathous – Having jaws that recede backwards.
phleg-	burn	**phleg**masia – Inflammation.
chem(o)	chemical	**chemo**therapy – Treatment of disease through the use of chemicals.
		chemosurgery – Use of chemicals to destroy diseased tissue.
-mittent	send	inter**mittent** – Alternating periods of activity and inactivity.
		re**mittent** – As of a fever with fluctuating body temperatures.
dips(o)	thirst	**dipso**gen – Something that induces thirst.
		dipsosis – Excessive thirst.
ped(o)	foot	**ped**icure – Professional treatment of the feet.
		pedograph – A footprint.
chord(o)	cord	**chord**ate – Having a notochord.
		chorditis – Inflammation of a vocal or spermatic cord.
onc(o)	tumor; barb	**onco**genesis – The growth of a tumor.
		oncovirus – A virus that produces a tumor.
		oncosphere – Tapeworm larvae within embryonic envelope and armed with six hooks.
cec(o)	cecum; blind	**cec**al – pertaining or associated with a blind passage; the cecum.
		cecitis – Inflammation of the cecum.
urethr(o)	urethra	**urethro**rrhagia – The flow of blood from the urethra.
		urethrostenosis – The narrowing of the urethra.

MEDICAL ROOTS / PREFIXES / SUFFIXES	MEANING	EXAMPLES
epi-	after; upon; in addition to	**epi**dural – Located on the dura mater.
		epidermis – The outer layer of skin.
dextr(o)	right (side)	ambi**dextro**us – Can use either hand well.
		dextrorotatory – Turning toward the right side.
sub-	under, beneath; below; inferior	**sub**cutaneous – Under the skin.
		sublingual – Beneath the tongue.
psamm(o)	sand	**psamm**oma – Any tumor containing psammoma bodies (round collections of calcium).
lig(o)	tie; bind	**lig**ase – An enzyme that joins together molecules.
		ligament – Tissue that connects bones or cartilage.
myx(o)	mucus	**myx**asthenia – A low secretion of mucus.
		myxadenitis – Inflammation of a mucous gland.
angi(o)	vessel	**angio**plasty – Surgical repair of blood vessels.
		angiography – Radiologic evaluation of blood vessels after injection of IV contrast dye.
dent(o)	tooth	**dent**algia – A toothache.
		dentist – A person who works on teeth.
phy(o)	produce; make	osteo**phy**ma – Tumor or outgrowth of a bone.
lymph(o)	lymph; water	**lymph**edema – Swelling caused by build up of lymph.
		lymphostasis – To stop the flow of lymph.

MEDICAL ROOTS / PREFIXES / SUFFIXES	MEANING	EXAMPLES
ecto-	outside	**ecto**derm – In a developing embryo, the outermost germ layer.
		ectopia – Displacement of an organ or body part from its normal position.
ichthy(o)	fish	**ichthy**osis – A disorder of the skin that causes scaliness, like fish skin.
		ichthyic – Pertaining to or like fish.
arthr(o)	joint	**arthr**algia – Pain of one or more joints.
		arthritis – Inflammation of one or more joints.
traum(a)	wound	**traum**atism – Physical or psychic state resulting from injury.
mening(o)	meninges; membrane	**meningo**malacia – Softening of a membrane.
		meningitis – Inflammation of the meninges.
-physis	growth	apo**physis** – An outgrowth. Often used to describe bony outgrowths that do not separate from the bone (e.g. tubercle process).
		sym**physis** – To grow together.
intra-	inside; within	**intra**venous – Inside a vein.
		intracellular – Within a cell or cells.
uter(o)	uterus; womb	**utero**pexy – Surgical fixation of the uterus.
		uteropelvic – Pertaining to the uterus and the pelvis.
gyr(o)	ring; circle	**gyr**ospasm – Spasm in which the head rotates around the neck.
		gyrate – Revolve around a fixed point.
meat(o)	course; passage	**meat**us – An opening or passage.
		meatotomy – Surgical incision of the urinary passage.
-porosis	porous; cavity formation	osteo**porosis** – A disease in which the bones are porous and fragile.

MEDICAL ROOTS / PREFIXES / SUFFIXES	MEANING	EXAMPLES
cervic(o)	neck; cervix (neck of the uterus)	**cervico**thoracic – Pertaining to the neck and thorax.
		cervicitis – Inflammation of the cervix of the uterus.
nulli-	none	**nulli**para – A woman who has never given birth to a child.
		nullify – To make void.
cerc(o)	tail	**cerc**aria – The larval form of a trematode worm whose body is terminated by a tail-like appendage.
		Hetero**cerc**al – In animals, a vertebral column continued into the upper lobe of the tail.
fasci(o)	band	**fasci**a – A sheet or band of fibrous tissue.
		fasciotomy – Surgical incision of a fascia.
sudor(i)	sweat	**sudor**iparous – To produce sweat.
labi(o)	lip	**labio**mental – Pertaining to the lip and chin.
		labiochorea – A spasm of the lips that interferes during speech.
mut(a)	mutation; change	**muta**gen – A substance that induces genetic mutation.
		mutase – An enzyme that changes chemical groups by shifting them from one position to another.
auto-	self	**auto**immunity – An immune response against tissues of the patient's own body.
		autotransfusion – Transfusion of the patient's own blood.
mi(o)	smaller; less	**mio**sis – Contraction of the pupil.
		miosphygmia – A condition in which there are fewer pulse beats than there are heart beats.

MEDICAL ROOTS / PREFIXES / SUFFIXES	MEANING	EXAMPLES
cost(o)	rib	**cost**algia – Pain in the ribs.
		inter**cost**al – Between the ribs.
helic(o)	coil	**helic**opod – A dragging gait.
		helical – Spiral.
loph(o)	tuft	**loph**otrichous – Having two or more flagella at one end.
sup-	under, beneath; below; inferior	**sup**pression – To hold back or stop.
		suppository – A medication that is inserted through lower openings such as the anus.
narc(o)	numb; stupor; sleep	**narco**lepsy – A disorder that causes uncontrolled episodes of deep sleep.
		narcosis – A sleep-like state.
prosop(o)	face	**prosopo**plegia – Paralysis of the face.
		prosoposchisis – Having a facial cleft.
intro-	within; into	**intro**spection – To look within.
		introvert – A person who keeps to themselves; to turn inward.
cheil(o)	lip	**cheilo**schisis – A split lip; harelip.
		cheilitis – Inflammation of the lips.
ambly(o)	dull	**ambly**aphia – Decreased sharpness of touch perception.
		amblyacousia – Decreased sharpness of hearing.
goni(o)	angle	**gonio**meter – An instrument used to measure angles.
		gonioscope – An instrument for examining the angular motion of the eye.
tyr(o)	cheese	**tyr**omatosis – Disease of caseous (resembling cheese) degeneration.

Conclusion

"If one advances confidently in the direction of his dreams and endeavors to live the life which he has imagined, he will meet with a success unexpected in common hours."

– Henry David Thoreau

CONCLUSION

By working through all medical combining forms, you have rightly placed a high level of importance on learning medical terminology. You should be commended on your perseverance and your effort will not go without reward. There is little doubt that the most efficient mechanism to prepare for any medical career is to become fluent in medical language. Rather than relying on the rote memorization of individual words, a solid knowledge of Greek and Latin combining forms allows you to break down complex terms into their components, permitting you to instantaneously deduce the meaning of words never seen before. The value and utility of this cannot be reiterated enough. The purpose of this chapter is to describe how the interactive website, **Medtutor.com**, can be used to master medical terminology.

The first priority is to continue studying combining forms until they are known well. The book is designed to be portable and can be easily carried during the course of the day, allowing for frequent, intermittent study as opportunity permits. The website contains interactive applications that can be used with conventional computers or mobile hand-held devices. The medical combining forms course includes applications that provide repeated exposure to these same combining forms in a fun and innovative format. The medical terminology course contains applications that go beyond the book by introducing thousands of new medical terms, the meanings of which can be deduced with a preexisting knowledge of combining forms.

The best way to learn is to be tested. Both the medical combining forms course and the medical terminology course are associated with a final comprehensive exam. Each exam should be approached in the same way a final exam in a formal course would and it is imperative not to take it until you are thoroughly prepared. Like the final exam of other *Medtutor* texts, you only get one opportunity to take each exam.

In order to take the comprehensive combining forms exam, you will need to go to the interactive website, **Medtutor.com**, and register. At this point, you will be granted 30 days of free access to the site if you were previously unregistered. During this time, you can further your study with the use of the interactive applications. If you wish to continue your subscription after 30 days, you may do so for a nominal subscription fee. Before taking the final exam, you should review all of the combining forms several times and participate in the web-based applications on a regular basis. Once you feel that you know them, schedule a particular date and time to take the exam. At least three hours of uninterrupted time should be set aside in order to complete it. Be sure to get plenty of sleep the night before and employ the rituals that have helped you with previous exams. The more you put into taking this exam, the greater the reward you attain.

The timed final exam consists of 180 questions displayed in a multiple choice format. The exam is administered in two ninety-minute segments and a break is permitted in-between them. The exam can seem long, but it is designed to mimic medical board exams in which mental fatigue often plays a role. At the conclusion of the test, you will immediately obtain a score and answers and detailed explanations are then provided. Every question is grouped into one of three categories (prefixes, suffixes, and word roots), so you will know how well you did in each category. You can also have the internet site send an e-mail that verifies your score to any individual, school, or admissions committee of your choosing.

As opposed to the terminal component of the course, the final exam should be viewed as a bridge to more advanced learning. Although you have already expended a substantial amount of effort to reach this point, it is imperative that you take the next step in your educational journey. The combining forms must be *known*, not just memorized long enough to get through the final exam. A solid knowledge of combining forms is the key that unlocks medical terminology. Repetitive exposure with use of the book and website will solidify your knowledge base.

Once you feel confident in your knowledge of combining forms, you can begin to utilize the internet applications of the medical terminology course. These applications allow the user to interpret and learn the meanings of previously unseen terms based on his or her preexisting knowledge of combining forms. The definition of each term is provided and the combining form components that are contained in the word are reviewed. The student obtains the dual benefit of developing an expertise in combining forms while also learning medical terminology. When ready, you can access and take the final exam of the terminology course. Because a letter of score certification can be e-mailed to individuals or organizations of your choosing, you should not take the final exam until thoroughly prepared.

The customizable web-based applications and training programs that compliment these courses include randomized exams, flashcards, and crossword puzzles. The website tracks the individual student's progress, allowing each student to tailor the exercises to focus on particular problem areas.

The **randomized exam system** includes a database of thousands of board-type questions. Those of the combining forms course are related to every combining form contained in this book. Each question is categorized to the type of combining form: prefixes, suffixes, and word roots. Each of the medical terminology questions is categorized to a specific medical specialty. Examples include general medicine, dentistry, cardiology, and orthopedics. The student can sporadically and repeatedly prompt the system to randomly assimilate a test of a desired number of questions. As directed by the student, this exam may contain questions specific to a particular combining form category and/or medical specialty, a group of categories and/or specialties, or even to a mixture of other *Medtutor* books and their chapters. Furthermore, the student can also direct the system to assemble exams solely from questions the student has never seen before, questions previously passed, questions previously failed, or a combination of all question categories. Problem areas can be identified and future work can be directed toward those areas.

To facilitate tracking, a progress bar and a score bar are provided for the pool of questions that are associated with each combining form category or medical specialty. This allows the student to instantaneously know where he or she currently stands within each category of information at any given time. Out of the total number of questions available for each category, the system displays the percentage of questions that have previously been answered by the student. This percentage is displayed as a *progress* bar. Out of the questions that have previously been answered, the system also displays the percentage that was answered correctly. This is displayed as a *score* bar. Like the final exam, each randomized exam is timed and graded upon completion. Detailed explanations are given and the student learns how well he or she did in the various categories. Upon completion of an exam, if so desired, the student can then direct the system to immediately create another randomized exam of desired specifications or participate in a different teaching application.

The **flashcard application** also possesses customizable properties that help the student manage information and learn. Thousands of flashcards are available and each is categorized to a particular type of combining form or medical specialty. Like the questions that appear in a randomized exam, flashcards may be studied based on a specific combining form category and/or medical specialty, a group of categories and/or specialties, or even to a mixture of other *Medtutor* books and book chapters. When requested by the user, an audio application can provide the correct pronunciation of terms that appear on the front of medical terminology flashcards.

At the completion of a particular set of cards, the student may prompt the system to display the same set of cards backwards in order to show the back of each card first. This reinforces recall and promotes learning. Alternatively, the student may direct the system to initially present the back of each card from the onset. The student has the ability to pass or fail him/herself on each flashcard. Failed flashcards are placed in a personalized databank that can be accessed at any time. With review, cards that are subsequently marked as "passed" are removed from this databank; "failed" cards remain.

The **medical crossword puzzles** constitute another innovative teaching application at **Medtutor.com**. The puzzles are an informal way to continually review and learn new material. As with other applications, the system can be directed to create a puzzle specific to information contained in the two courses associated with this book or some combination of other *Medtutor* courses. If the answer to a crossword question is not known, the application provides a short explanation when requested. Crossword puzzles can be worked online or printed and worked while away from the computer. The student can return to the internet site to check answers and obtain explanations. Once a puzzle is completed, the system can immediately create a new puzzle as directed by the student. Among other utilities, the medical crossword puzzle application is a fun and effective means to consistently review and maintain a tangible knowledge base long after the texts are finished. There is a significant amount of fundamental medical information presented in the *Medtutor* series; even working just one puzzle a day would greatly benefit any practitioner in a health-related profession.

Other *Medtutor* courses are available at **Medtutor.com**. The goal of each is to provide a system that is convenient and conducive to a lifetime of learning. The texts provide information in an easy to understand format and the web-based applications give a recreational and repetitive exposure to the medical facts. Health-related careers can be very challenging and the more information a practitioner knows, the higher the quality of care he or she can provide. If you don't use it, you lose it and the *Medtutor* courses are designed to help you both learn and maintain your knowledge in the most efficient way possible.